Alveolar Bone Grafting Techniques for Dental Implant Preparation

Guest Editor

PETER D. WAITE, MPH, DDS, MD

ORAL AND MAXILLOFACIAL SURGERY CLINICS OF NORTH AMERICA

www.oralmaxsurgery.theclinics.com

Consulting Editor
RICHARD H. HAUG, DDS

August 2010 • Volume 22 • Number 3

SAUNDERS an imprint of ELSEVIER, Inc.

W.B. SAUNDERS COMPANY
A Division of Elsevier Inc.

1600 John F. Kennedy Blvd. ● Suite 1800 ● Philadelphia, PA 19103-2899

www.oralmaxsurgery.theclinics.com

ORAL AND MAXILLOFACIAL SURGERY CLINICS OF NORTH AMERICA Volume 22, Number 3
August 2010 ISSN 1042-3699, ISBN-13: 978-1-4377-2472-1

Editor: John Vassallo; j.vassallo@elsevier.com
Developmental Editor: Donald Mumford

Oral and Maxillofacial Surgery Clinics of North America (ISSN 1042-3699) is published quarterly by Elsevier Inc., 360 Park Avenue South, New York, NY 10010-1710. Months of issue are February, May, August, and November. Business and Editorial Offices: 1600 John F. Kennedy Blvd., Suite 1800, Philadelphia, PA 19103-2899. Periodicals postage paid at New York, NY and additional mailing offices. Subscription prices are $304.00 per year for US individuals, $445.00 per year for US institutions, $140.00 per year for US students and residents, $351.00 per year for Canadian individuals, $530.00 per year for Canadian institutions, $405.00 per year for international individuals, $530.00 per year for international institutions and $190.00 per year for Canadian and foreign students/residents. To receive student/resident rate, orders must be accompanied by name or affiliated institution, date of term, and the *signature* of program/residency coordinator on institution letterhead. Orders will be billed at individual rate until proof of status is received. Foreign air speed delivery is included in all *Clinics* subscription prices. All prices are subject to change without notice. **POSTMASTER:** Send address changes to *Oral and Maxillofacial Surgery Clinics of North America,* Elsevier Periodicals Customer Service, 11830 Westline Industrial Drive, St. Louis, MO 63146. Tel: 1-800-654-2452 (U.S. and Canada); 314-447-8871 (outside U.S. and Canada). Fax: 314-447-8029. E-mail: journalscustomerservice-usa@elsevier.com (for print support); journalsonlinesupport-usa@elsevier.com (for online support).

Reprints. For copies of 100 or more, of articles in this publication, please contact the Commercial Reprints Department, Elsevier Inc., 360 Park Avenue South, New York, NY 10010-1710. Tel.: 212-633-3812; Fax: 212-462-1935; Email: reprints@elsevier.com.

Oral and Maxillofacial Surgery Clinics of North America is covered in MEDLINE/PubMed (*Index Medicus*).

Printed and bound in the United Kingdom
Transferred to Digital Print 2011

Contributors

CONSULTING EDITOR

RICHARD H. HAUG, DDS
Carolinas Center for Oral Health
Charlotte, North Carolina

GUEST EDITOR

PETER D. WAITE, MPH, DDS, MD
Professor and Chair, Department of Oral and
Maxillofacial Surgery, University of Alabama
School of Dentistry, University of Alabama at
Birmingham, Birmingham, Alabama

AUTHORS

RUTH APONTE-WESSON, DDS, MS
Associate Professor and Professor,
Department of Prosthodontics, School
of Dentistry, University of Alabama
at Birmingham, Birmingham, Alabama

WILLIAM BELL, DDS
Professor, Department of Oral and Maxillofacial
Surgery and Pharmacology, Baylor College
of Dentistry, Dallas, Texas

ARTURO BILBAO, MD, PhD
Department of Oral and Maxillofacial Surgery,
Santiago de Compostela University Hospital;
Private Practice, Santiago de Compostela, Spain

HAIYAN CHEN, PhD
Instructor, Department of Oral and Maxillofacial
Surgery; Institute of Oral Health Research,
School of Dentistry, University of Alabama
at Birmingham, Birmingham, Alabama

JARED COTTAM, DDS, MD
Implant Dentistry Associates of Colorado,
Oral and Maxillofacial Surgery, Greenwood
Village, Colorado

JOSEPH DEATHERAGE, DMD, MD
Department of Oral and Maxillofacial Surgery,
University of Alabama at Birmingham,
Birmingham, Alabama

NICOLAAS C. GEURS, DDS, MS
Associate Professor, Department
of Periodontology, University of Alabama
at Birmingham, Birmingham, Alabama

FARAH Y. GHORI, MD
Institute of Oral Health Research, School
of Dentistry, University of Alabama
at Birmingham, Birmingham, Alabama

RAJESH GUTTA, BDS, MS
Assistant Professor, Department of Oral and
Maxillofacial Surgery, University of Texas
Health Science Center, San Antonio, Texas

JON D. HOLMES, DMD, MD, FACS
Private Practice, Oral and Facial Surgery
of Alabama; Clinical Assistant Professor,
Department of Oral and Maxillofacial Surgery,
University of Alabama at Birmingham,
Birmingham, Alabama

AMJAD JAVED, MSc, PhD
Associate Professor of Oral and Maxillofacial
Surgery, Cell Biology and Molecular Pathology,
School of Dentistry, University of Alabama
at Birmingham, Birmingham, Alabama

OLE T. JENSEN, DDS, MS
Implant Dentistry Associates of Colorado,
Oral and Maxillofacial Surgery, Greenwood
Village, Colorado

JACK E. LEMONS, PhD
University Professor, Departments
of Prosthodontics, Surgery and Biomedical
Engineering, Schools of Dentistry, Medicine
and Engineering, University of Alabama
at Birmingham, Birmingham, Alabama

PATRICK J. LOUIS, DDS, MD
Professor and Residency Program Director,
Department of Oral and Maxillofacial Surgery,
University of Alabama at Birmingham,
Birmingham, Alabama

MICHAEL S. REDDY, DMD, DMSc
Professor and Chair, Department of
Periodontology, University of Alabama
at Birmingham, Birmingham, Alabama

R. DAVID RODEN JR, DMD, MD
Burton and Roden Oral and Maxillofacial Surgery,
Birmingham, Alabama

SOMSAK SITTITAVORNWONG, DDS, MS, DMD
Assistant Professor, Department of Oral and
Maxillofacial Surgery, University of Alabama
at Birmingham, Birmingham, Alabama

PHILIP J. VASSILOPOULOS, DDS
Assistant Professor, Department of
Periodontology, University of Alabama
at Birmingham, Birmingham, Alabama

LUIS G. VEGA, DDS
Assistant Program Director, Oral and
Maxillofacial Residency Program and Assistant
Professor, Division of Oral and Maxillofacial
Surgery, Department of Surgery, Health Science
Center at Jacksonville, University of Florida,
Jacksonville, Florida

KENNETH J. ZOUHARY, DDS, MD
Chief, Department of Oral and Maxillofacial
Surgery, Birmingham Veterans Affairs Medical
Center; Assistant Professor, University of Alabama
Oral and Facial Surgery, Birmingham, Alabama

Contents

Genetic and Transcriptional Control of Bone Formation   283

Amjad Javed, Haiyan Chen, and Farah Y. Ghori

> An exquisite interplay of developmental cues, transcription factors, and coregulatory and signaling proteins support formation of skeletal elements of the jaw during embryogenesis and dynamic remodeling of alveolar bone in postnatal life. These molecules promote initial condensation of the mesenchyme, commitment of the mesenchymal progenitor to osteogenic lineage cells, and differentiation of committed osteoblasts to mature osteocytes within mineralized bone. Parallel regulatory networks promote formation of the functional osteoclast from mononuclear cells to support continuous bone remodeling within the alveolar bone. With an ever expanding list of new regulatory factors, the complexities of the molecular mechanisms that control gene expression in skeletal cells are being further appreciated. This article examines the multifunctional roles of prominent nuclear proteins, cytokines, hormones, and paracrine factors that control osteogenesis.

Principles of Bone Grafting   295

R. David Roden Jr

> This article reviews the principles of bone healing and bone grafting. There are many different ways to reach the same goal when bone grafting procedures are performed. With all of the available methods and materials, a clear understanding of these basic principles will assist in the selection of a technique for each individual patient.

Bone Graft Harvesting From Distant Sites: Concepts and Techniques   301

Kenneth J. Zouhary

> Bony augmentation of the moderately to severely resorbed alveolus in preparation for endosseous dental implant placement can be challenging for the oral and maxillofacial surgeon. Autogenous bone remains the gold standard for alveolar grafting. Multiple extraoral bone graft sources can be used to help meet this challenge, including the iliac crest, proximal tibia, and calvarium. This article reviews the anatomy, harvest techniques, and morbidity associated with each of these donor sites.

Bone Graft Harvesting from Regional Sites   317

Somsak Sittitavornwong and Rajesh Gutta

> Bone grafts are widely used in the reconstruction of osseous defects in the oral and maxillofacial region. Successful osseointegration of dental implants requires sufficient bone surrounding the implant. Although bone substitutes and augmentation techniques offer viable prognoses for achieving the required amount of hard tissue augmentation, autologous bone is the gold standard with regard to quantity, quality, and an uneventful healing. Autogenous bone grafts are generally obtained from the ilium, the

rib, and the calvarium. Alternative sources for local harvesting in the mandible can be evaluated by careful clinical and radiographic examinations of the patient. This article discusses the various sources of grafts and the techniques used to harvest bone.

This article focuses on the emergence of the small edentulous osteoperiosteal flap.

The restoration of bony defects has followed an interesting course through history. From the early use of animal materials to bone grown in the laboratory, the goal of restoring bony defects has generated ingenuity in solving these significant clinical challenges.

With tooth loss, there is increased bone loss of the alveolus. In some cases alveolar bone loss can be severe. Severe bone loss may cause difficulty for patients wearing a conventional prosthesis or being restored with dental implants. Severe alveolar bone loss can result in malnutrition, poor self-esteem, multiple dental visits for failed prosthesis, and jaw fracture. In many cases, patients with loss of alveolar bone height or width may require reconstructive procedures. Vertical ridge augmentation remains a challenge in the reconstruction of the atrophic maxilla and mandible. The main problem arises from the need to expand the soft-tissue envelope and achieve the proper bony architecture. Techniques that have been developed to solve or circumvent this problem include onlay bone grafting with particulate bone graft, block bone graft, barrier techniques with permanent or resorbable membranes, distraction osteogenesis, vascularized ridge splitting techniques, sinus lifts, nerve repositioning techniques, short implants, and angled implants. All of these techniques have advantages and disadvantages. This article focuses on augmentation procedures using titanium mesh, which acts as a barrier and physical support of the soft tissue over the bone graft.

Alveolar distraction is a constantly evolving technique. A review of the literature within the past 14 years reveals that there are clear indications for its use, with outcomes similar to and sometimes even more predictable than traditional bone grafting techniques in preparation for implant placement. Although complications exist with alveolar distraction, it seems that most are minor and easy to manage. Appropriate patient selection and a better understanding of the technique are paramount to successful bone regeneration with alveolar distraction osteogenesis. This article discusses newer research and provides clinical advice on the practice of alveolar distraction osteogenesis for dental implant preparation.

Healthy soft tissue surrounding a dental implant is essential for health, function, and esthetics. The development of the tooth includes the formation of a biologic connection between the living tissues that has to be created during the healing process after placement of the implant. The success of dental implants is dependent on the establishment of a soft-tissue barrier that is able to shelter the underlying osseous structures and the osseointegration surrounding the implant body. The esthetics of a dental implant prosthesis depends on the health and stability of the peri-implant mucosa. Understanding of soft-tissue healing and maintenance around dental implants is paramount for implant success. This article discusses the soft-tissue interface, aspects of soft-tissue health, and esthetics during treatment planning and therapy.

The transfer of composite tissue flaps by microvascular techniques has become the standard for reconstructing complex defects of the oral and maxillofacial regions. Despite advances in these techniques, sites reconstructed by free tissue transfer (free flaps) are often compromised by scarring, bulky tissue, and altered architecture. Dental rehabilitation is often impossible without endosseous implants to aid in stabilization and retention of prostheses. The most commonly used free flaps, however, have significant shortcomings with regard to implant placement, prosthetics, and maintenance. This article describes some site development and prosthetic techniques that can be applied to improve outcomes when dental implants are used in conjunction with free flap reconstruction.

This article briefly explains the process of, and provides examples from, dental surgical implant device retrieval and analysis. Study results of three areas where unique and new information has been or is being published within professional journals are summarized. An analysis of past and current activities strongly supports opportunities for more in-depth investigations of explanted and postmortem-type specimens. It seems that these types of protocols will be supportive of more fully investigating the clinical applications for successful and unsuccessful outcomes of evolving tissue-engineered medical products as alternatives to some types of synthetic-origin implant devices.

Oral and Maxillofacial Surgery Clinics of North America

THE CLINICS ARE NOW AVAILABLE ONLINE!

Access your subscription at:
www.theclinics.com

Preface
Alveolar Bone Grafting Techniques for Dental Implant Preparation

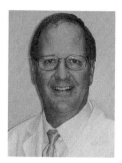

Peter D. Waite, MPH, DDS, MD
Guest Editor

Bone grafting for implant site preparation has become a new surgical technique niche similar to what preprosthetic surgery was for removable dentures. Preprosthetic surgery is almost a lost art, but the surgical techniques necessary for alveolar reconstruction or implant site preparation have become much more complex and variable. The surgical art of ridge reconstruction in preparation for dental implants in many ways has become more important and complex than the simple placement of dental implants. The final prosthetic result depends on creating the correct alveolar arch morphology, alignment, and symmetry. Oral and maxillofacial surgeons (OMSs) are best trained to address this unique surgical niche.

Bone grafting techniques are not new for the OMS, and therefore basic principles used in alveolar cleft grafting and jaw reconstruction after trauma and oncologic defects are valuable clinical applications. However, bone grafting for implant patients are quite different in many ways. Such patients often expect minimal morbidity, outpatient clinic procedures, and reasonable private financing. The amount of bone required is much less, but the stability and predictability much higher. We now know that just getting an implant in bone is not adequate if the biologic width and soft tissue is insufficient. Cosmetic reconstruction begins with the correct alveolar bone height and contour. The role of the OMS in the dental implant team will become more important as the public comes to expect natural cosmetic, long-term

stability. Much of what we do is pragmatic, and dogma changes from year to year, or speaker to speaker.

The purpose of this issue is to lay out a logical approach to alveolar reconstruction and bone grafting for implant preparation. This begins with the basic science of bone biochemistry and physiology. In recent years, we have come to understand bone at a much deeper level. Understanding the human genome has unlocked some of the secrets that regulate bone deposition and resorption. Although the first article may be partially incomprehensible for the surgeon, it is important to know that bone products are developing with sound scientific structure. Bone is a much more dynamic matrix with multiple regulating factors than previously thought. It is exciting to discuss clinical problems with our basic science colleagues and share in the translational research. Basic science understanding does change the surgeon's behavior. The principles of bone grafting are applicable for the simple socket graft, sandwich graft, or the sinus lift. We must establish minimally invasive office-based procedures that yield predictable outcomes. Bone must be harvested by predictable surgical techniques, whether from local or distant sites. The OMSs are trained to harvest the best bone indicated, and therefore choice is not limited to just allogenic bone (bottle bone). New procedures such as ridge splitting, distraction osteogenesis, and titanium mesh are examples of this new surgical niche

Oral Maxillofacial Surg Clin N Am 22 (2010) ix–x
doi:10.1016/j.coms.2010.06.004

oralmaxsurgery.theclinics.com

that are built on the solid surgical principles of the past. No bone graft or surgical procedure will be successful without adequate vasculature and soft tissue protection. We learn most from our failures, and the article on explantation gives us valuable information on the biomaterials of implants.

I hope our specialty finds this issue to be a valuable contribution to the clinical practice of preimplant surgery. I have learned a great deal by editing the articles, and it has already changed my surgical approach and techniques. I want to thank each of the authors who worked so hard over and beyond their normal duties to make this issue possible.

Peter D. Waite, MPH, DDS, MD
Department of Oral and Maxillofacial Surgery
University of Alabama School of Dentistry
University of Alabama at Birmingham
419 School of Dentistry Building
1530 3rd Avenue South
Birmingham, AL 35294-0007, USA

E-mail address:
pwaite@uab.edu

Genetic and Transcriptional Control of Bone Formation

Amjad Javed, MSc, PhD[a],*, Haiyan Chen, PhD[a],
Farah Y. Ghori, MD[b]

KEYWORDS

- Bone development • Skeletal remodeling • Osteoblast
- Molecular signaling

Skeletogenesis in mammals requires coordinated activities of multiple cell types and is formed by two distinct developmental processes.

1. Endochondral ossification: Most skeletal elements in the body, including all long bones, are derived by this process. Sequential maturation and degradation of a chondrocyte-produced cartilaginous template is a prerequisite for osteoblast recruitment. The second step in endochondral ossification is the eventual replacement of cartilage matrix with mineralized matrix synthesized by osteoblasts.
2. Intramembranous ossification: Craniofacial skeletal elements are primarily derived through this process whereby cells in condensed mesenchyme directly differentiate into mineralizing osteoblasts.

DEVELOPMENTAL ORIGIN OF ALVEOLAR BONE

During embryonic development, blocks of condensed mesenchyme are modeled into precisely shaped cartilaginous elements.[1] In humans, this process of skeletal patterning is completed within the first trimester of pregnancy (ninth week after conception). Subsequently, the skeletal tissue template undergoes a dramatic increase in size and ossification but with a relatively small change in the basic shape of bones. In mammals, the mandibular and maxillary bones develop from the first branchial arch during embryonic skeletal patterning.[2] The alveolar bone and processes in the maxilla and mandible are formed by intramembranous ossification. However, cellular components of the craniofacial skeleton are unique and include cranial neural crest-derived ectomesenchyme.[3,4] The mandibular and maxillary alveolar process houses and supports the dentition. Tooth development initiates as a local thickening of oral epithelium that subsequently grows into the underlying neural crest-derived mesenchyme of the first branchial arch.[5,6] Tooth development proceeds through multiple stages of differentiation that are morphologically distinct, such as dental lamina, bud, cap, bell, crown, and root. In human deciduous teeth, formation of dental lamina is noted within 7 weeks of gestation, with the ultimate cytodifferentiation of odontoblasts that

This work was supported by Grant No. RO1 AG030228 from the National Institutes of Health.

[a] Department of Oral and Maxillofacial Surgery, School of Dentistry, University of Alabama at Birmingham, Birmingham, AL, USA

[b] Institute of Oral Health Research, School of Dentistry, University of Alabama at Birmingham, SDB 713, 1530 3rd Avenue South, Birmingham, AL 35294-0007, USA

* Corresponding author. Institute of Oral Health Research, University of Alabama at Birmingham, SDB 714, 1530 3rd Avenue South, Birmingham, AL 35294-0007.

E-mail address: javeda@uab.edu

produce the dentin extracellular matrix (ECM) within 18 weeks. Although the alveolar bone is formed in relation to the teeth, structurally it is similar to the basal bone and alveolar bone cells closely resemble skeletal osteoblasts.[3]

OSTEOBLAST BIOLOGY

During embryonic development, osteoblasts originate from local mesenchyme and, postnatally, from bone marrow stromal stem cells or connective tissue mesenchymal stem cells (MSCs). In response to specific stimuli, these precursor cells commit to osteogenic lineage and differentiate into mature osteoblasts. Extensive research in the past 20 years by many laboratories have defined the sequence of events that results in the maturation of osteoblasts.[7–13] Distinct osteoblast stages that are characterized by the expression of specific genes and functional properties have been established using in vitro cell culture and in vivo models and by determining modifications in gene expression in normal and pathological bone tissues. Profiles of gene expression in vivo further define the substages of osteoblast maturation, and these substages are altered as a result of genetic mutations.

In general, osteoblastogenesis is defined by four major phases: lineage commitment, proliferative expansion, synthesis of the ECM, and mineralization. All these stages are characterized by sequentially expressed genes that support the progression of osteoblastic differentiation through developmental transition points (**Fig. 1**). The first transition requires MSC commitment to osteogenic lineage; the second is associated with mitotic duplication and expansion of osteoprogenitor; the third requires exit from the cell cycle and robust production of the ECM by osteoblasts; and the final stage is marked by mineralization of the ECM and establishment of osteocytes.

Self-renewing MSCs are pluripotent and can give rise to multiple tissue-type lineages, such as osteoblast, odontoblastic, chondrocyte, myoblast, adipocyte, and tendon cell. However, the MSCs and osteoprogenitors are not readily identifiable, because of the lack of distinct morphologic features and histochemical markers. Initially, the Stro-1 antibody was used to isolate the adherent population from adult bone marrow cells, but the surface antigen is ubiquitously expressed.[14] Recent reports show that a combination of multiple cell surface markers and absence of hematopoietic stem cell lineage markers significantly enrich MSC population from bone marrow. However, so far, no single specific marker has been identified that can select and enrich osteoprogenitors from all tissues.

The first step in development of the osteoblast phenotype is lineage commitment and formation of osteoprogenitors. This commitment is regulated by master transcription factors and their coregulators. This step involves expression of lineage-inducing factors and inhibition of factors that maintain lineage plasticity. The key factors for commitment of osteogenic cell type include Runx2, Osterix, Sox9, and morphogens, transforming growth factor β (TGFβ)/ bone morphogenetic proteins (BMPs), and fibroblast growth factors (FGFs). The initial progenitors are still bipotential and can commit to osteo- or chondro-lineage depending on the threshold of Sox and Runx2/Osterix. Vitamin D3, glucocorticoids, parathyroid hormone, and estrogen are shown to regulate parameters of the proliferation/growth in a dosage- and time-dependent fashion.[15–20] These hormones and cytokines influence the progression of MSCs into osteoblast lineage, directly or indirectly, by suppressing signaling that promotes commitment to other lineages, such, as adipocyte and myoblast.[21,22]

In the second stage of osteoblast development, there is extensive proliferation of progenitor cells with expression of growth-related genes (histones, c-myc, and c-fos). The proliferation stage encompasses a wide range of osteogenic cell types, from the pluripotent MSC to the more committed chondro-osteoprogenitor and preosteoblast. During this proliferative phase, several matrix genes begin to be expressed (eg, type I collagen, fibronectin, and some growth factors such as BMP2/TGFβ). Transcription factors that support proliferation of multipotential MSCs also suppress phenotypic genes that are usually induced at the postproliferative stage of osteoblast differentiation, such as helix-loop-helix factors (HLH), Twist, Groucho/TLE, and Id. These transcription factors maintain proliferating progenitor cells in an undifferentiated state.[9,23]

The third stage of osteoblast differentiation corresponds to a period of osteoblasts clustering and multilayering in cultures and the synthesis and maturation of the ECM. This stage is characterized by the expression of alkaline phosphatase, an early marker of the postproliferative osteoblast phenotype, and production of a collagen matrix. The accumulation of type I collagen ECM initiates marked reduction in histone expression, an exit from the cell cycle, and the cessation of cell proliferation. Moreover, collagen ECM promotes the signaling cascade by cell-matrix and cell-cell interactions to support the expression of osteoblast-related genes.[24–27] During this stage,

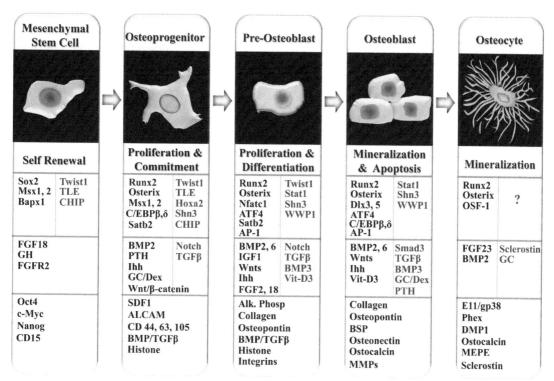

Mesenchymal Stem Cell		Osteoprogenitor		Pre-Osteoblast		Osteoblast		Osteocyte	
Self Renewal		Proliferation & Commitment		Proliferation & Differentiation		Mineralization & Apoptosis		Mineralization	
Sox2	Twist1	Runx2	Twist1	Runx2	Twist1	Runx2	Stat1	Runx2	
Msx1, 2	TLE	Osterix	TLE	Osterix	Stat1	Osterix	Shn3	Osterix	?
Bapx1	CHIP	Msx1, 2	Hoxa2	Nfatc1	Shn3	Dlx3, 5	WWP1	OSF-1	
		C/EBPβ,δ	Shn3	ATF4	WWP1	ATF4			
		Satb2	CHIP	Satb2		C/EBPβ,δ			
				AP-1		AP-1			
FGF18		BMP2	Notch	BMP2, 6	Notch	BMP2, 6	Smad3	FGF23	Sclerostin
GH		PTH	TGFβ	IGF1	TGFβ	Wnts	TGFβ	BMP2	GC
FGFR2		Ihh		Wnts	BMP3	Ihh	BMP3		
		GC/Dex		Ihh	Vit-D3	Vit-D3	GC/Dex		
		Wnt/β-catenin		FGF2, 18			PTH		
Oct4		SDF1		Alk. Phosp		Collagen		E11/gp38	
c-Myc		ALCAM		Collagen		Osteopontin		Phex	
Nanog		CD 44, 63, 105		Osteopontin		BSP		DMP1	
CD15		BMP/TGFβ		BMP/TGFβ		Osteonectin		Ostcalcin	
		Histone		Histone		Osteocalcin		MEPE	
				Integrins		MMPs		Sclerostin	

Fig. 1. Ontogeny of osteoblasts and regulatory control of osteoblast lineage progression and phenotypic features. Sequence and stages of the osteoblast lineage from a self-renewing, pluripotent MSC to a terminally differentiated osteocyte are diagrammatically illustrated. The characteristic feature of each developmental stage is indicated below the cell morphology. Next row summarizes the key transcription factor and coregulatory protein involved in genetic control of osteoblast differentiation. Factors that negatively regulate Runx2 activity and osteoblast differentiation are indicated in red. Several physiologic mediators influencing osteoblast development are also indicated, including transforming growth factor β (TGFβ), bone morphogenetic proteins (BMPs), fibroblast growth factors (FGFs), Wnt/β-Catenin signaling, and hormones. Secretory molecules, receptor, and signal transducer that inhibit osteoblast maturation are highlighted in red. Last row summarizes phenotypic marker genes expressed at different developmental stages of osteoblast differentiation.

the maximal levels of collagen synthesis and assembly is coupled with induction of noncollagenous ECM proteins, such as osteopontin, osteonectin, bone sialoprotein, and osteocalcin.[9]

The final stage of osteoblastogenesis is characterized by deposition of minerals in the ECM, concomitant with peak expression of genes considered markers of the mature osteoblast.[28–31] These include but are not limited to bone sialoprotein, osteocalcin, and osteopontin. This phase begins with down-regulation of matrix-maturing proteins and robust expression of gene products associated with the mineralization that leads to formation and accumulation of hydroxyapatite crystals. During this period, marked morphologic changes are evident in vivo, with transition of some cuboidal osteoblasts to fibroblast-looking lining cells or the stellate osteocyte (see **Fig. 1**). Most osteoblasts (approximately 85%) do not achieve the end-stage phenotype of an osteocyte and undergo programmed cell death. Apoptotic

osteoblasts show increased expression of Bad and Bax genes, and matrix-degrading enzymes and suppression of Bcl2, a pro-cell survival gene.[32–34] Osteocytes are spatially and morphologically distinct from osteoblasts, because they are completely encased in bone and possess dendritic processes. The long-branched cellular processes allow them to contact each other as well as osteoblasts and lining cells present on the bone surface and marrow stromal cells on the endosteum. Some of the genes considered markers of mature osteoblasts are also expressed in osteocytes (osteocalcin, MEPE, DMP1). However, in recent years, a few signature genes of osteocytes, such as E11/gp38, Phex, and sclerostin, have been identified.[35] It is estimated that there are ten thousand osteocytes per cubic millimeter of bone, and about 50 dendritic processes are present on each cell.[36] Therefore, osteocytes make up more than 90% to 95% of the cellular component of the adult skeleton compared with

4% to 6% of osteoblasts and only 1% to 2% of osteoclasts. The long-lived osteocytes function as the mechanosensors of skeletal tissues.[35]

Profiles of differentially expressed genes and their responses to physiologic cues have provided an important conceptual framework for defining distinct stages of osteoblast maturation and cellular understanding of bone development and bone remodeling.

Stem Cells, MSCs, and Induced Pluripotent Stem Cells

Unlike pluripotent embryonic stem (ES) cells, the stem cells derived from postnatal tissues are multipotent. They self-renew through potent proliferative capacity and can give rise to at least two types of highly differentiated lineages.[37] Various adult tissues contain reservoirs of specific stem cells that support maintenance and regeneration of the parental tissue. The ever-expanding list of tissues containing specific stem cells include epidermis and intestinal crypts for epithelial stem cells, brain neural tissues for neural stem cells, skeletal muscle with satellite stem cells, and several connective tissues for MSCs.[37–40]

Historically, the adult bone marrow has been used as a source of different types of stem cells, such as hematopoietic stem cells and MSCs, because of convenient isolation.[41] The marrow-derived MSCs are capable of differentiating into mesenchymal (bone, cartilage, muscle, tendon, adipose, and other connective tissues) and non-mesenchymal tissues in vitro and in vivo.[37–40] The progeny of MSCs are responsible for postnatal bone formation and adult fracture repair and remodeling.

Commitment and differentiation of these cells to bone, cartilage, tendon, ligament, and muscle lineage is a complex process involving multiple discrete cellular transitions. Progression from one stage to the next requires the presence of specific bioactive factors and dynamic environmental cues whose exquisitely controlled contributions orchestrate the differentiation program.[9,11] MSCs have been successfully purified and expanded in invitro culture from both animals and humans. The relative ease of isolation, in vitro mitotic expansion, and multi-lineage differentiation as well as their autologous nature are key to the emergence of human MSCs as a potential source of cell-based therapy for genetic disorders and for reconstruction and bone tissue engineering. However, the widespread use of MSCs for the treatment of many clinically challenging conditions is hampered by their limited supply and significant loss of differentiation capacity in long-term cultures.

Cellular differentiation and lineage commitment are considered to be robust and irreversible processes during development. The diverse cell types present in the adult organism are produced by ES cells during development by lineage-specific transcription factors. This has fueled attempts to study the transcriptional circuitry that controls pluripotency and self-renewal of ES cells. The master regulators and signaling pathways of ES cell population are beginning to be identified.[42] A cocktail of four transcription factors that can induce pluripotency and promote and maintain the undifferentiated state of mouse and human adult somatic cells has recently been characterized.[42] This approach using induced pluripotent stem (iPS) cells would allow maintenance of phenotypic plasticity, ex vivo expansion, and directed differentiation of MSCs or osteoprogenitor population for use in tissue engineering and reconstruction of bone tissues. Human iPS cells produced by expression of Oct4, Sox2, c-Myc, and Klf4 or by Oct4, Sox2, Nanog, and Lin28 are remarkably similar to human ES cells. Being morphologically similar as well, they express typical human ES cell-specific cell surface antigens and genes, differentiate into multiple lineages in vitro, and form teratomas containing differentiated derivatives of all three primary germ layers when injected into immunocompromised mice.[43]

More importantly, iPS cells can be derived from skin cells of patients with various diseases and without c-Myc oncogene and viral integration.[43–45] These discoveries eliminate a major roadblock for developing customized iPS cells tailored to patient-specific needs, and translating theraputic usage of these cells. Although these specific factors are sufficient for induced pluripotency, it is still unclear how these genes orchestrate the erasure of the differentiated state and cause lineage reprogramming of adult somatic cells.

The use of iPS technology is not imminent, but the ability to produce stem cells by induced pluripotency has provided therapeutic options that have never been available. This has also rekindled hopes of treating generalized conditions like osteoporosis by systemic administration of culture-expanded autologous iPS cells/MSCs or repairing local bone defects through site-directed delivery of reprogrammed cells.

Transcriptional Regulation of Osteoblast Differentiation

Aided by combined developmental, molecular, genetic, biochemical, and cellular approaches, transcriptional regulation is the most actively investigated area of bone research. Osteoblast commitment, differentiation, and functional activity are all governed by several regulatory proteins and specific transcription factors that promote expression of phenotypic genes and establishment of the osteoblast phenotype. The recent development of molecular genetic studies in human skeletal pathobiology coupled with genetic mouse models have contributed to a better understanding of the regulatory machinery involved in the control of osteoblastogenesis.[7–10] The role of key signaling molecules, transcription factors, and chromatin remodeling enzymes that control the formation and maturation of osteoblasts are summarized.

Regulatory factors that influence various aspects of osteoblast biology can be divided into four major categories. These include (1) *cis*-acting DNA binding transcription factors, (2) signal transducers and non-DNA binding coregulatory proteins, (3) posttranslational regulatory proteins, and (4) chromatin-modifying enzymes. Regulatory factors in the last 2 categories are functional through all stages of osteoblast differentiation; however, their target genes and proteins are restricted to a specific stage of osteoblastic differentiation.

Two transcription factors that are predominantly expressed in osteoblasts are obligatory for commitment of mesenchymal progenitors to osteoblast lineage and for development of the functional osteoblast. The first protein, Runx2, is a member of the runt domain family of transcription factors and regulates various aspects of osteoblastic biology.[8,9] Developmentally, Runx2 expression is first noted in osteochondroprogenitor cells of the condensing mesenchyme at the onset of skeletal development. Levels of Runx2 gradually increase in subsequent stages of osteoblastic differentiation, with maximum expression observed in the mature osteoblast. Runx2 gene deletion in mice results in complete absence of bone formation and failure of osteoblast and chondrocyte maturation.[46] Consistently in humans, Runx2 haploinsufficiency results in cleidocranial dysplasia, a disease characterized by defective bone formation and supernumerary teeth.[47] Runx2 is both necessary and sufficient for mesenchymal cell differentiation toward osteoblast lineage, because Runx2 overexpression can convert mesenchymal cells of other lineages to the osteogenic phenotype and Runx2 inhibition blocks the differentiation of mesenchymal cells to osteoblasts.[48] Runx2 controls bone lineage cells by binding to the Runx regulatory element in promoters of genes considered to be markers for different stages of osteoblastic differentiation.[9,49] Runx2 target genes include those expressed by immature and differentiated osteoblasts, such as TGF-β receptor, alkaline phosphatase, collagen type I α_1 and α_2 chain, osteopontin, osteonectin, Vitamin D receptor, galectin-3, bone sialoprotein, osteocalcin, and collagenase.[9]

The second DNA-binding transcription factor that is absolutely required for osteoblast differentiation is Osterix. Osterix/SP7 is a member of the zinc-finger containing SP family and is abundantly expressed throughout osteoblast differentiation.[50] Genetic inactivation of Osterix in mice results in absence of mineralized bone matrix, defective osteoblasts, and perinatal lethality.[50] Similar to Runx2, forced expression of Osterix in nonbone cells promotes expression of early and late stage marker genes of osteoblasts. However, molecular and genetic studies revealed that Runx2 is expressed in mesenchymal tissues of Osterix-null mice.[50] Thus, Osterix acts downstream of Runx2 in the transcriptional cascade of osteoblast differentiation. Consistently, Osterix expression is positively regulated by direct binding of Runx2 to a responsive element in the promoter of the Osterix gene.

Multiple transcription factors that are expressed ubiquitously also play a critical role in bone homeostasis and development of functional osteoblasts. This group consists of proteins that bind DNA in a sequence-specific manner and those that do not directly interact with the DNA, such as CCAAT/enhancer-binding proteins (C/EBPs), ATF4, NFATc, AP-1, Dlx5, Smads, CBFβ, and Satb2.[51–55] They regulate osteoblast differentiation by directly inducing the expression of target genes and/or by modulating the activities of Runx2 and Osterix transcription factors. For example, ATF4 and C/EBPs induce expression of osteoblastic genes through direct binding to their respective *cis*-element in the promoters.[52,53] Both proteins also form a physical complex with Runx2 to synergistically regulate the transcription of osteocalcin. Therefore, disruption of ATF4 or C/EBP genes in mice results in delayed skeletal development, decreased bone formation, and osteopenia phenotype.[53] Similarly, Osterix is shown to interact physically and functionally with NFATc to induce osteoblast gene expression, and NFATc deficiency causes a severe low–bone-mass phenotype because of decreased bone formation.[56] The list of transcription factors that function as coactivators of Runx2 is rapidly growing and includes AP-1, Dlx3, Dlx5, Menin, Smads, and TAZ.[9]

Examples of non-DNA binding proteins that cooperatively regulate Runx2-dependent osteoblast differentiation include Satb2 and Cbfβ. Satb2 is the nuclear matrix protein with affinity for the matrix attachment regions of chromatin loops. Satb2 physically interacts with Runx2 and ATF4 to enhance their promoter occupancy and with the transcriptional function of Runx2 to regulate osteocalcin expression and promote osteoblast differentiation. Satb2-null mice have defective craniofacial bones because of inhibited osteoblast differentiation.[55] All members of the Runx family of proteins usually interact with CBFβ cofactor through the runt domain. CBFβ does not directly interact with DNA but enhances the DNA-binding affinity of Runx2 severalfold, leading to the increased functional competency of Runx2.[54] Consistent with this notion, CBFβ deletion affects skeletal development and osteoblast maturation.[54]

Runx2-mediated commitment of mesenchymal cells to osteoblast lineage is also supported by homeodomain-containing transcription factors Bapx1 and Msx2. Both proteins act upstream of Runx2 in a transcriptional cascade that regulates osteoblast differentiation. Accordingly, Msx2- and Bapx1-deficient mice display severe dysplasia of the ossified skeleton and a strong reduction in expression of Runx2 in early mesenchymal progenitor cells.[57]

As a master transcriptional regulator, Runx2 is capable of activating and repressing expression of multiple genes required for the progression of osteoblast differentiation. Runx2 functional activity is suppressed actively during early stages of mesenchymal cell commitment toward osteoblast lineage by Groucho/TLE, Stat1, and Twist. The Groucho/TLE and Twist proteins are expressed early during skeletogenesis and in mesenchymal progenitors. Twist proteins prevent Runx2 protein from binding target-gene DNA by physically associating with the DNA-binding domain of the Runx2 protein.[58] In contrast, TLE protein inhibits Runx2 transcriptional activity by interacting with the C-terminal transcriptional activation domain.[59] Dramatic decreases in expression of the Twist and TLE genes result in relieving Runx2 inhibition and progression of osteoblast differentiation. Stat1 transcription factor inhibits Runx2 function during osteoblast differentiation by preventing nuclear import of Runx2. Stat1 interaction with Runx2 results in cytoplasmic sequestration of Runx2.[60] Enhanced bone formation seen in Stat1-deficient mice is linked to robust nuclear translocation of Runx2 and increased osteoblast differentiation.

Post-translational modification of Runx2 that results in ubiquitination-mediated degradation is another mechanism by which osteoblast differentiation is regulated. Runx2 interacts with enzymes responsible for protein stability, such as Shn3, WWP1, Smurf1, and CHIP.[61,62] Smurf1 was the first factor identified as an E3 ligase for Runx2 ubiquitination and degradation. Similarly, Schnurri 3, a zinc-finger adaptor protein in osteoblasts, links Runx2 to the E3 ubiquitin ligase WW domain-containing protein 1. These interactions initiate proteasomal degradation of Runx2.[61] Runx2 protein is stabilized in Shn3-deficient osteoblasts and Shn3-null mice shows severe increase in bone mass.[61] CHIP, a cochaperone protein identified recently promotes the ubiquitination and degradation of chaperone-bound proteins. CHIP interacts with Runx2 in vitro and in vivo and regulates Runx2 protein stability.[62] Decrease in CHIP expression results in a concomitant increase in Runx2 protein and osteoblastic differentiation.[62]

The ability of Runx2 to activate or repress transcription of multiple genes required for the progression of osteoblast differentiation is regulated through chromatin modification of the target gene promoter.[9] Transcriptional activity is dependent on the state of chromatin condensation, and histone modifications that decondense chromatin facilitate recruitment of transcription factors and expression. Runx2 directly interacts and recruits p300 acetyltransferase and histone deacetylase to regulate osteoblast genes.[9,63]

Thus Runx2, Osterix, and associated regulatory protein complexes are important for directing mesenchymal precursor cells toward osteoblast lineage.

Regulation of Osteoblast Differentiation by Secreted Molecules

Spatiotemporal organization of the osteoprogenitors in developing bones and the multiple stages of osteoblast differentiation are regulated by coordinated expression of a complex series of signaling molecules and associated transcription factors. Skeletal cells produce numerous growth factors and cytokines that signal in auto- and paracrine fashion to control cell proliferation, differentiation, and survival. These secreted factors and signaling pathways promote or suppress the expression and/or function of transcription factors essential for osteoblast differentiation. The major pathways involved in skeletal morphogenesis and development of the osteoblast phenotype include members of the FGF, TGFβ, and hedgehog families, Wnt signaling, and notch pathway.

The FGF pathway consists of 23 ligands that transduce their signal through one of the four FGF receptors (FGFRs). FGFs initiate condensation of the mesenchyme and proliferation of progenitor cells. Temporal expression and the activity of FGFRs are critical for membranous bone formation and regulate the proliferation, differentiation, and apoptosis of osteoblasts.[64] FGFRs contribute to normal skeletal development, because mutation or gene deletions are associated with severe dwarfism.[65] FGF ligands such as 2, 3, 4, 9, and 18 are associated with normal skeletal development; mutation or gene deletion in these is associated with skeletal deformities and delayed suture closure.[65] FGF-18 plays a critical role in maturation of osteoblasts and FGF-2 increases Runx2 phosphorylation and functional activity.[66] Similarly, activation of FGFR2 signaling triggers increased Runx2 expression and enhanced osteoblast differentiation.[66]

The widely known secreted molecules with potent capacity to induce osteogenesis are the BMPs. BMPs are members of the TGFβ superfamily of growth factors, which are produced by almost all skeletal cell types and induce mesenchymal condensations for the formation of many organs and skeleton patterning.[67] BMPs signal through homomeric or heteromeric type I and type II receptors, which are expressed in all cell types including osteoblasts. Specific BMP receptors influence lineage direction. Stimulation of mesenchymal progenitor cells by BMP2 dramatically induces expression of Runx2 and Osterix, leading to osteoblastic differentiation.[9,51,68] Induction of Runx2 and Osterix by BMP2 and subsequent upregulation of osteoblast-specific genes involves Dlx5, Smad transducers, and mitogen-activated protein kinase (MAPK) pathway. Although BMPs, when applied locally, induce de novo bone formation by recapitulating osteoblast differentiation, not all fall into this category. For example, BMP3 strongly inhibits osteoblast differentiation and proliferation.[69] TGFβ plays a complex role during bone remodeling, with inhibition of Runx2 and osteoblast differentiation in vitro but promotion of bone formation in vivo.[9,67,70]

Wnt proteins have emerged as central regulators of bone synthesis and bone mass. The canonical pathway that works through intracellular transducer β-Catenin controls differentiation of osteoblast progenitor cells into mature osteoblasts. β-Catenin is expressed in mesenchymal precursor cells and its inactivation favors their differentiation into chondrocytes instead of osteoblasts.[71] In human receptor mutations that render a constitutively active Wnt signal, results in a generalized increase of bone mass throughout the skeleton.[72] Wnt signaling controls osteoblast differentiation by modulating several transcription factors, including Runx2. Wnt signaling promotes Runx2 expression and activity. LEF/TCF transcription factors, the end point of the Wnt signal in the nucleus, promote Runx2 and Osterix expression and interact with Runx2 to regulate its function during osteoblast differentiation.[73]

Indian hedgehog (Ihh), a secreted molecule of the hedgehog family is widely known for its role in chondrocytes during endochondral bone formation.[74] Ihh and its receptor are also expressed in osteoblasts. Mice in which the Ihh gene is deleted lack osteoblast progenitor cells.[74] Ihh is also needed for osteoblast proliferation and survival. It controls osteoblast differentiation, first, by inducing expression of Runx2 in mesenchymal cells and second, by enhancing osteogenic action of Runx2 through an interaction between signal transducer Gli2 and Runx2 in osteoblasts.[75]

Notch receptors are the latest addition to the signaling molecules vital for osteoblast differentiation and bone remodeling. Notch signaling requires cell-cell interaction between the four Notch receptors and their ligands present on the cell surface. In humans, mutations in Notch signaling cause skeletal patterning defects. Notch-deficient mice develop severe osteoporosis.[76] Notch inhibits osteoblast differentiation by physically associating with Runx2 and interfering with its functional activity. Through its expression in osteoblasts, Notch exerts a dimorphic effect during bone remodeling. Notch inhibits osteoclast differentiation by controlling production of decoy-receptor osteoprotegerin by osteoblasts.[76]

Although several hormones regulate osteoblastic differentiation and influence bone formation and bone remodeling, we will briefly review two hormones responsible for regulating calcium metabolism. Parathyroid hormone (PTH) produced by the chief cells of the parathyroid gland plays a central role in calcium homeostasis through its action on bone and kidney and through enhanced synthesis of another hypercalcemic hormone, 1,25(OH)2 vitamin D3.[77] The capacity of exogenous PTH to function as an anabolic agent depends on direct and indirect stimulation of cells of osteoblast lineage. PTH promotes bone formation partly through phosphorylation and activation of Runx2, resulting in expression of osteoblast genes.[78] PTH also inhibits proteasome-mediated degradation of Runx2 and increases expression of osterix to enhance osteoprogenitor lineage determination.[79] Another regulatory action of PTH is to promote the β-Catenin pathway, which controls osteoblast survival.[80] Thus, PTH regulates bone development, bone maturation, and bone maintenance through the regulation of Runx2 function.

The other major hypercalcemic hormone, 1,25(OH)2 vitamin D3, is a steroid hormone that favors intestinal absorption of calcium.[81] Deletion or inactivation of the vitamin D receptor (VDR) in mice and in humans leads to rickets, a phenotype partially reversible in both organisms by treatment with calcium. Vitamin D3 positively regulates the expression of osteoblast phenotypic markers.

REMODELING OF ALVEOLAR BONE

During replacement of the primary dentition with permanent teeth, the alveolar bone undergoes a complete remodeling. The alveolar bone associated with the primary tooth is completely resorbed together with the roots of the tooth while new alveolar bone is formed to support the newly erupted tooth.[82] Significant remodeling of the alveolar process also occurs as part of this process. The ability of the alveolar bone to remodel rapidly also facilitates positional adaptation of teeth in response to functional forces and the physiologic drift of teeth that occurs with the development of jaw bones.[82]

Bone remodeling involves the coordination of activities of cells from two distinct lineages, the bone-synthesizing osteoblasts and the bone-resorbing osteoclasts. Each step in the remodeling process is regulated by specific hormones, local factors, and mechanical forces. Osteoclasts, the exclusive bone resorptive cells, are derived from the bone marrow macrophage lineage, but osteoblasts are required for their differentiation. Macrophage colony stimulating factor (M-CSF) and receptor activator nuclear factor-κB ligand (RANKL), the two cytokines produced by osteoblasts, are essential and sufficient for osteoclastogenesis.[83] These soluble proteins are produced by mesenchymal progenitors in marrow and osteoblasts. M-CSF contributes to the proliferation, survival, and differentiation of osteoclastic precursors and the survival and cytoskeletal rearrangement required for efficient bone resorption. Formation of macrophage requires an interaction of the M-CSF ligand with the receptor present on the surface of the mononuclear precursor. The M-CSF–receptor interaction also induces the expression of RANK on the surface of macrophage.[83] The second cytokine produced by osteoblasts is RANKL. Once linked to its receptor, RANK, on the surface of macrophage, it induces their fusion and differentiation. Thus, the bone microenvironment is essential for two components of osteoclastogenesis: (1) maturation and fusion of the mononuclear precursor to the multinucleated osteoclast and (2) regulation of the activity of the functional osteoclast.

Osteoblasts also produces osteoprotegerin (OPG), a high-affinity ligand and physiologic inhibitor of RANKL.[84] OPG is secreted by cells of mesenchymal origin basically and in response to other regulatory signals including cytokines and bone-targeting steroids. Proinflammatory cytokines suppress OPG expression while simultaneously enhancing that of RANKL, the net effect being a marked increase in osteoclast formation and function. Thus, circulating OPG modulates the bone resorptive activity of RANKL. Gene deletion of OPG in humans and mice leads to profound osteopetrosis, whereas overexpression of OPG results in severe osteoporosis.

Prostaglandins are another factor that influence bone mass. Prostaglandin excess stimulates bone loss by increasing expression of RANKL and suppressing that of OPG in stromal and osteoblastic cells.[85] This increase in OPG/RANKL ratio is sufficient for increased osteoclastic activity. Therefore, the balance between RANKL and OPG determines the formation and activity of osteoclasts.

Sex steroids are central to maintenance of bone mass and bone remodeling. This action indirectly relates to regulation of the production of multiple cytokines by different cell types in the bone marrow microenvironment. Estrogen mediates its effect by suppression of cytokines that are involved in the regulation of osteoclast formation. For example, estrogen inhibits production of interleukin(IL) -1 and tumor necrosis factor α (TNF-α) by monocytes and IL-6, granulocyte macrophage (GM)-CSF, and M-CSF by osteoblasts.[86] Estrogen can also suppress osteoclastogenesis by enhanced production of OPG and decreased RANKL production by osteoblasts.[87] Similarly, testosterone is shown to decrease osteoclast formation and resorption through increased production of OPG by osteoblasts.[88] Thus osteoprogenitors and osteoblasts are essential regulators of the cellular and molecular events involved in bone remodeling.

SUMMARY

Bone is crucial to the human body, providing skeletal support and serving as a home for the formation of hematopoietic cells and a reservoir for calcium and phosphate. Over time, an understanding has grown of how large numbers of morphogens, signaling molecules, and transcriptional regulators form the complex tissue of bone. Key factors regulating the gene expression program that underlies the induction, proliferation, differentiation, and maturation of osteoblasts are presented here. Secreted growth factors and hormones determine the competency of osteoblasts for establishing and maintaining the structural and functional properties of bone. It is increasingly clear that these diverse transcription factors cannot be viewed as discrete signaling pathways; rather, they form a highly interconnected, cooperative network to allow progression of osteoblast differentiation. Bone is also continuously remodeled by hematopoietic lineage osteoclasts. Osteoblast-produced factors are essential regulators of osteoclast differentiation and their bone resorbing function. A better understanding of molecular mechanisms behind osteogenic differentiation and bone remodeling helps to identify pathogenic causes of bone and skeletal diseases and leads to the development of targeted therapies for these diseases.

REFERENCES

1. Shubin NH, Alberch PA. Morphogenic approach to the origin and basic organization of the tetrapod limb. Evol Biol 1986;20:319–87.
2. Osumi-Yamashita N, Ninomiya Y, Eto K, et al. The contribution of both forebrain and midbrain crest cells to the mesenchyme in the frontonasal mass of mouse embryos. Dev Biol 1994;164(2):409–19.
3. Sodek J, McKee MD. Molecular and cellular biology of alveolar bone. Periodontol 2000 2000;24:99–126.
4. Zernik JH, Nowroozi N, Liu YH, et al. Development, maturation, and aging of the alveolar bone. New insights. Dent Clin North Am 1997;41(1):1–15.
5. Chai Y, Jiang X, Ito Y, et al. Fate of the mammalian cranial neural crest during tooth and mandibular morphogenesis. Development 2000;127:1671–9.
6. Thesleff I, Aberg T. Molecular regulation of tooth development. Bone 1999;25(1):123–5.
7. Ducy P, Schinke T, Karsenty G. The osteoblast: a sophisticated fibroblast under central surveillance. Science 2000;289(5484):1501–4.
8. Karsenty G. Transcriptional control of skeletogenesis. Annu Rev Genomics Hum Genet 2008;9:183–96.
9. Lian JB, Javed A, Zaidi SK, et al. Regulatory controls for osteoblast growth and differentiation: role of Runx/Cbfa/AML factors. Crit Rev Eukaryot Gene Expr 2004;14(1–2):1–41.
10. Stein GS, Lian JB. Molecular mechanisms mediating proliferation/differentiation interrelationships during progressive development of the osteoblast phenotype. Endocr Rev 1993;14(4):424–42.
11. Aubin JE. Regulation of osteoblast formation and function. Rev Endocr Metab Disord 2001;2(1):81–94.
12. de Crombrugghe B, Lefebvre V, Nakashima K. Regulatory mechanisms in the pathways of cartilage and bone formation. Curr Opin Cell Biol 2001;13(6):721–7.
13. Karsenty G, Kronenberg HM, Settembre C. Genetic control of bone formation. Annu Rev Cell Dev Biol 2009;25:629–48.
14. Gronthos S, Zannettino AC, Graves SE, et al. Differential cell surface expression of the STRO-1 and alkaline phosphatase antigens on discrete developmental stages in primary cultures of human bone cells. J Bone Miner Res 1999;14(1):47–56.
15. Canalis E, Delany AM. Mechanisms of glucocorticoid action in bone. Ann N Y Acad Sci 2002;966:73–81.
16. Nijweide PJ, Burger EH, Feyen JH. Cells of bone: proliferation, differentiation, and hormonal regulation. Physiol Rev 1986;66(4):855–86.
17. Suda T, Udagawa N, Nakamura I, et al. Modulation of osteoclast differentiation by local factors. Bone 1995;17(Suppl 2):87S–91S.
18. Kronenberg HM. PTHrP and skeletal development. Ann N Y Acad Sci 2006;1068:1–13.
19. Jilka RL, O'Brien CA, Ali AA, et al. Intermittent PTH stimulates periosteal bone formation by actions on post-mitotic preosteoblasts. Bone 2009;44(2):275–86.
20. Parfitt AM. Parathyroid hormone and periosteal bone expansion. J Bone Miner Res 2002;17(10):1741–3.
21. Kato S, Suzawa M, Takada I, et al. The function of nuclear receptors in bone tissues. J Bone Miner Metab 2003;21(6):323–36.
22. Canalis E. Update in new anabolic therapies for osteoporosis. J Clin Endocrinol Metab 2010;95(4):1496–504.
23. Jensen ED, Gopalakrishnan R, Westendorf JJ. Regulation of gene expression in osteoblasts. Biofactors 2010;36(1):25–32.
24. Damsky CH. Extracellular matrix-integrin interactions in osteoblast function and tissue remodeling. Bone 1999;25(1):95–6.
25. Franceschi RT, Xiao G. Regulation of the osteoblast-specific transcription factor, Runx2: responsiveness to multiple signal transduction pathways. J Cell Biochem 2003;88(3):446–54.
26. Stupack DG, Cheresh DA. Get a ligand, get a life: integrins, signaling and cell survival. J Cell Sci 2002;115(Pt 19):3729–38.
27. Cheresh DA, Stupack DG. Integrin-mediated death: an explanation of the integrin-knockout phenotype? Nat Med 2002;8(3):193–4.
28. Boskey AL, Wright TM, Blank RD. Collagen and bone strength. J Bone Miner Res 1999;14(3):330–5.
29. Glimcher MJ. Mechanism of calcification: role of collagen fibrils and collagen-phosphoprotein complexes in vitro and in vivo. Anat Rec 1989;224(2):139–53.
30. Gericke A, Qin C, Sun Y, et al. Different forms of DMP1 play distinct roles in mineralization. J Dent Res 2010;89(4):355–9.
31. Robey PG. Bone proteoglycans and glycoproteins. In: Bilezikian JP, Raisz LA, Rodan GA, editors. Principal of bone biology. San Diego (CA): Academic Press; 2002. p. 225–38.

32. Xing L, Boyce BF. Regulation of apoptosis in osteo-clasts and osteoblast cells. Biochem Biophys Res Commun 2005;328(3):709–20.

33. Jilka RL, Weinstein RS, Bellido T, et al. Osteoblast programmed cell death (apoptosis): modulation by growth factors and cytokines. J Bone Miner Res 1998;13(5):793–802.

34. Lynch MP, Capparelli C, Stein JL, et al. Apoptosis during bone-like tissue development in vitro. J Cell Biochem 1998;68(1):31–49.

35. Dallas SL, Bonewald LF. Dynamics of the transition from osteoblast to osteocyte. Ann N Y Acad Sci 2010;1192(1):437–43.

36. Bonewald LF, Johnson ML. Osteocytes, mecha-nosensing and Wnt signaling. Bone 2008;42(4):606–15.

37. Watt FM, Hogan BL. Out of Eden: stem cells and their niches. Science 2000;287(5457):1427–30.

38. Slack JM. Stem cells in epithelial tissues. Science 2000;287:1431–3.

39. McKay R. Stem cells in the central nervous system. Science 1997;276:66–71.

40. da Silva Meirelles L, Nardi NB. Murine marrow-derived mesenchymal stem cell: isolation, in vitro expansion, and characterization. Br J Haematol 2003;123:702–11.

41. Wagers AJ, Weissman IL. Plasticity of adult stem cells. Cell 2004;116:639–48.

42. Graf T, Enver T. Forcing cells to change lineages. Nature 2009;462(7273):587–94.

43. Belmonte JC, Ellis J, Hochedlinger K, et al. Induced pluripotent stem cells and reprogramming: seeing the science through the hype. Nat Rev Genet 2009;10(12):878–83.

44. Ebert AD, Yu J, Rose FF Jr, et al. Induced pluripotent stem cells from a spinal muscular atrophy patient. Nature 2009;457:277–80.

45. Lee G, Papapetrou EP, Kim H, et al. Modelling patho-genesis and treatment of familial dysautonomia using patient-specific iPSCs. Nature 2009;461:402–6.

46. Komori T, Yagi H, Nomura S, et al. Targeted disrup-tion of Cbfa1 results in a complete lack of bone formation owing to maturational arrest of osteo-blasts. Cell 1997;89:755–64.

47. Mundlos S, Otto F, Mundlos C, et al. Mutations involving the transcription factor CBFA1 cause clei-docranial dysplasia. Cell 1997;89:773–9.

48. Ducy P, Zhang R, Geoffroy V, et al. Osf2/Cbfa1: a transcriptional activator of osteoblast differentia-tion. Cell 1997;89:747–54.

49. Javed A, Gutierrez S, Montecino M, et al. Multiple Cbfa/AML sites in the rat osteocalcin promoter are required for basal and vitamin D-responsive tran-scription and contribute to chromatin organization. Mol Cell Biol 1999;19(11):7491–500.

50. Nakashima K, Zhou X, Kunkel G, et al. The novel zinc finger-containing transcription factor osterix is required for osteoblast differentiation and bone formation. Cell 2002;108:17–29.

51. Javed A, Bae JS, Afzal F, et al. Structural coupling of Smad and Runx2 for execution of the BMP2 osteo-genic signal. J Biol Chem 2008;283(13):8412–22.

52. Gutierrez S, Javed A, Tennant DK, et al. CCAAT/ enhancer-binding proteins (C/EBP) beta and delta activate osteocalcin gene transcription and syner-gize with Runx2 at the C/EBP element to regulate bone-specific expression. J Biol Chem 2002; 277(2):1316–23.

53. Yang X, Matsuda K, Bialek P, et al. ATF4 is a substrate of RSK2 and an essential regulator of osteoblast biology; implication for Coffin-Lowry Syndrome. Cell 2004;117:387–98.

54. Kundu M, Javed A, Jeon JP, et al. Cbfbeta interacts with Runx2 and has a critical role in bone develop-ment. Nat Genet 2002;32(4):639–44.

55. Dobreva G, Chahrour M, Dautzenberg M, et al. SATB2 is a multifunctional determinant of craniofacial patterning and osteoblast differentiation. Cell 2006; 125:971–86.

56. Koga T, Matsui Y, Asagiri M, et al. NFAT and Osterix cooperatively regulate bone formation. Nat Med 2005;11:880–5.

57. Tribioli C, Lufkin T. The murine Bapx1 homeobox gene plays a critical role in embryonic development of the axial skeleton and spleen. Development 1999; 126:5699–711.

58. Bialek P, Kern B, Yang X, et al. A twist code deter-mines the onset of osteoblast differentiation. Dev Cell 2004;6:423–35.

59. Javed A, Guo B, Hiebert S, et al. Groucho/TLE/R-esp proteins associate with the nuclear matrix and repress RUNX (CBF(alpha)/AML/PEBP2(alpha)) dependent activation of tissue-specific gene tran-scription. J Cell Sci 2000;113(Pt 12):2221–31.

60. Kim S, Koga T, Isobe M, et al. Stat1 functions as a cytoplasmic attenuator of Runx2 in the transcrip-tional program of osteoblast differentiation. Genes Dev 2003;17:1979–91.

61. Jones DC, Wein MN, Oukka M, et al. Regulation of adult bone mass by the zinc finger adapter protein Schnurri-3. Science 2006;312:1223–7.

62. Li X, Huang M, Zheng H, et al. CHIP promotes Runx2 degradation and negatively regulates osteo-blast differentiation. J Cell Biol 2008;181(6):959–72.

63. Vega RB, Matsuda K, Oh J, et al. Histone deacety-lase 4 controls chondrocyte hypertrophy during skeletogenesis. Cell 2004;119(4):555–66.

64. Ornitz DM, Marie PJ. FGF signaling pathways in endochondral and intramembranous bone develop-ment and human genetic disease. Genes Dev 2002; 16(12):1446–65.

65. Liu Z, Xu J, Colvin JS, et al. Coordination of chondro-genesis and osteogenesis by fibroblast growth factor 18. Genes Dev 2002;16:859–69.

66. Kim HJ, Kim JH, Bae SC, et al. The protein kinase C pathway plays a central role in the fibroblast growth factor-stimulated expression and transactivation activity of Runx2. J Biol Chem 2003;278(1):319–26.

67. Wu X, Shi W, Cao X. Multiplicity of BMP signaling in skeletal development. Ann N Y Acad Sci 2007;1116: 29–49.

68. Celil AB, Campbell PG. BMP-2 and insulin-like growth factor-I mediate Osterix (Osx) expression in human mesenchymal stem cells via the MAPK and protein kinase D signaling pathways. J Biol Chem 2005;280(36):31353–9.

69. Daluiski A, Engstrand T, Bahamonde ME, et al. Bone morphogenetic protein-3 is a negative regulator of bone density. Nat Genet 2001;27:84–8.

70. Kang JS, Alliston T, Delston R, et al. Repression of Runx2 function by TGF-beta through recruitment of class II histone deacetylases by Smad3. EMBO J 2005;24(14):2543–55.

71. Day TF, Guo X, Garrett-Beal L, et al. Wnt/beta-catenin signaling in mesenchymal progenitors controls osteoblast and chondrocyte differentiation during vertebrate skeletogenesis. Dev Cell 2005;8: 739–50.

72. Boyden LM, Mao J, Belsky J, et al. High bone density due to a mutation in LDL-receptor-related protein 5. N Engl J Med 2002;346:1513–21.

73. Bennett CN, Longo KA, Wright WS, et al. Regulation of osteoblastogenesis and bone mass by Wnt10b. Proc Natl Acad Sci U S A 2005;102(9):3324–9.

74. Maeda Y, Nakamura E, Nguyen MT, et al. Indian hedgehog produced by postnatal chondrocytes is essential for maintaining a growth plate and trabecular bone. Proc Natl Acad Sci U S A 2007;104:6382–7.

75. Shimoyama A, Wada M, Ikeda F, et al. Ihh/Gli2 signaling promotes osteoblast differentiation by regulating Runx2 expression and function. Mol Biol Cell 2007;18(7):2411–8.

76. Hilton MJ, Tu X, Wu X, et al. Notch signaling maintains bone marrow mesenchymal progenitors by suppressing osteoblast differentiation. Nat Med 2008;14:306–14.

77. Chorev M, Rosenblatt M. Parathyroid hormone: structure-function relations and analog design. In: Bilezikian JP, Raisz LG, Rodan GA, editors. Principles of bone biology. San Diego (CA): Academic Press; 1996. p. 305–23.

78. Krishnan V, Moore TL, Ma YL, et al. Parathyroid hormone bone anabolic action requires Cbfa1/Runx2-dependent signaling. Mol Endocrinol 2003; 17(3):423–35.

79. Bellido T, Ali AA, Plotkin LI, et al. Proteasomal degradation of Runx2 shortens parathyroid hormone-induced anti-apoptotic signaling in osteoblasts. A putative explanation for why intermittent administration is needed for bone anabolism. J Biol Chem 2003;278(50):50259–72.

80. Tobimatsu T, Kaji H, Sowa H, et al. Parathyroid hormone increases beta-catenin levels through Smad3 in mouse osteoblast cells. Endocrinology 2006;147(5):2583–90.

81. Dusso AS, Brown AJ. Mechanism of vitamin D action and its regulation. Am J Kidney Dis 1998;32:S13–24.

82. Sodek J. A comparison of the rates of synthesis and turnover of collagen and non-collagen proteins in adult rat periodontal tissues and skin using a microassay. Arch Oral Biol 1977;22:655–65.

83. Boyle WJ, Simonet WS, Lacey DL. Osteoclast differentiation and activation. Nature 2003;423:337–42.

84. Simonet WS, Lacey DL, Dunstan CR, et al. Osteoprotegerin: a novel secreted protein involved in the regulation of bone density. Cell 1997;89:309–19.

85. Kobayashi T, Narumiya S. Function of prostanoid receptors: studies on knockout mice. Prostaglandins Other Lipid Mediat 2002;68-69:557–73.

86. Riggs BL. The mechanisms of estrogen regulation of bone resorption. J Clin Invest 2000;106(10):1203–4.

87. Michael H, Härkönen PL, Väänänen HK, et al. Estrogen and testosterone use different cellular pathways to inhibit osteoclastogenesis and bone resorption. J Bone Miner Res 2005;20(12):2224–32.

88. Chen Q, Kaji H, Kanatani M, et al. Testosterone increases osteoprotegerin mRNA expression in mouse osteoblast cells. Horm Metab Res 2004; 36(10):674–8.

Principles of Bone Grafting

R. David Roden Jr, DMD, MD

KEYWORDS

• Bone grafting • Osteocytes • Osteoclasts • Fibroblasts

The maxilla and the mandible are embryologically derived from the first branchial arch. They both have a cartilage scaffold during development, but unlike bones of the appendicular skeleton, these cartilages only act as a scaffold for neural crest cells to form the bone. This type of bone formation is known as intramembranous ossification and is similarly found in the calvarium and other facial bones. The appendicular bones arise from preformed cartilage. Under the direction of regulatory proteins, neural crest cells migrate along the cartilaginous scaffolds of the maxilla and mandible to begin the process of bone formation.[1]

Bone is classified as cortical bone and trabecular bone between the cortices. Cortical bone is made of dense, compact bone containing series of haversian systems with lacunae housing osteocytes. Trabecular bone fills the marrow space between the cortices. This bone consists of series of trabeculae and is also known as spongy bone. Cells in the trabecular bone include osteoblasts, osteoclasts, and hematopoietic cells.

BONE HISTOLOGY

Histologically, compact bone is divided into multiple osteons or haversian systems, the functional units of bone. Each osteon has a central haversian canal containing vasculature. Volkmann canals are present allowing for biochemical communication between osteons. Osteocytes are housed in lacunae and communicate with each other through series of canaliculi. Osteocytes are terminally differentiated osteoblasts and are the primary mechanoreceptors of bone. There is evidence that osteocytes function as the regulator of bone turnover by monitoring fluid flow through their processes in the canalicular system.[2]

Trabecular bone houses the cells responsible for bone turnover and regeneration. Osteoblasts are the cells responsible for bone formation. They arise from osteoprogenitor cells. They are found in the trabecular bone as well as on the inner surface of the periosteum lining the outer surface of the cortical bone. Osteoblasts produce osteoid, the matrix for bone formation, made primarily of type 1 collagen. Once osteoblasts are surrounded by the matrix they produce, they further differentiate into osteocytes and no longer produce matrix.

Osteoclasts are cells responsible for bone resorption. They start out as mononucleated precursor cells in the macrophage linage and through a series of signals become activated multinucleated osteoclasts. Once in the marrow, osteoclasts, through delicate hormonal regulation, resorb bone. The process of resorption creates ruffled edges and forms Howship's lacunae where the osteoclast is housed.

BONE MEMBRANES

The cells responsible for the osteogenic potential of bone are housed in the tissues lining bone. The outer layer, periosteum, contains osteoblasts and progenitor cells in its inner surface or cambium layer. The lining of the internal surface of the bone, endosteum, also contains osteoblasts and osteoprogenitor cells.

BONE MATRIX

Bone consists of both organic and inorganic substances. The organic part of bone constitutes approximately 30% of bone and is 90% type 1 collagen. The remaining 10% of organic bone is comprised of noncollagen proteins. Sixty-five to

Burton and Roden Oral and Maxillofacial Surgery, 1771 Independence Ct, Suite 2, Birmingham, AL 35216, USA
E-mail address: audavid1@hotmail.com

Oral Maxillofacial Surg Clin N Am 22 (2010) 295–300
doi:10.1016/j.coms.2010.06.001

oralmaxsurgery.theclinics.com

seventy percent of bone is inorganic and made up primarily of hydroxyapatite $(Ca_{10}[PO_4]_6[OH]_2)$. Other minerals present in the inorganic part of bone include magnesium, potassium, chlorine, iron, and carbonate. Cortical bone can be differentiated from cancellous bone by the orientation of the collagenous matrix.

BONE HEALING

Bone healing can be subclassified into primary and secondary healing. As with soft tissue healing, primary healing of bone implies direct contact or a gap of less than 1 mm between bone fragments. This process of healing occurs by osteoclasts working in groups to create a cutting cone. Following this cutting cone of osteoclasts are osteoblasts secreting osteoid for future mineralization.

Secondary bone healing occurs through formation of a callus within which osteoid is produced and mineralization occurs. This type of bone healing can be divided into three major phases. The first phase is the inflammatory phase, which occurs immediately. There is formation of a hematoma, which eventually becomes granulation tissue. The repair stage then begins as inflammatory cells and fibroblasts invade the tissue. These cells cause differentiation and recruitment of osteoblasts and provide a scaffold for further vascular ingrowth. The osteoblasts lay down osteoid and form the soft callus. This callus eventually is ossified. The final stage of healing occurs with remodeling. This phase occurs over months to years and restores the bone to its original shape and near its original strength.

The principles of primary and secondary bone healing can be applied to bone graft healing. The type of graft material used, block versus particulate, dictates which healing process occurs.

Cortical block bone grafts heal by a process called creeping substitution. This process is similar to primary bone healing. Once the nonvascularized graft material is transferred to the defect, osteoclasts begin to resorb the graft material, allowing for fibroblast ingrowth and the creation of a matrix for vascularization of the graft. The osteoclasts create voids in the graft material that are filled with osteoid from osteoblasts. This osteoid then becomes mineralized. Once the graft material is resorbed, the newly formed bone undergoes remodeling and maturation. Ideally, the grafted bone would be completely resorbed, and new bone would be formed. The cortical block graft is never fully resorbed and replaced by new bone. The grafted bone remains as necrotic centers mixed with the newly formed bone.

Particulate, cortical, or cancellous, bone grafts begin the healing process by apposition of bone. They provide the necessary scaffold for ingrowth of osteoblasts and precursor cells into the defect. This apposition of bone is followed by resorption of the graft material. Ideally, there is complete resorption of the graft material, which is replaced by mature bone. Because cancellous grafts do not have to first undergo resorption before apposition, they revascularize faster than cortical block grafts. There is a much higher percentage of newly formed bone and greater resorption of the graft material when particulate grafts are used.

Autogenous cancellous marrow grafts undergo a well-documented and predictable healing process.[3] Transferred in the graft are osteocompetent marrow stem cells and osteoblasts. These cells initially survive at the grafted site through plasmatic diffusion of oxygen and nutrients. During week 1, platelets degranulate and release growth factors that are chemotactic, mitogenic, and angiogenic. These growth factors include:

PDGFaa
PDGFbb
PDGFab
TGF-β1
TGF-β2
VEGF
EGF.

During weeks 2 and 3, the graft is undergoing revascularization through capillary ingrowth. As revascularization occurs, the osteoblasts are induced to synthesize osteoid. Osteoid synthesis and secretion occurs during weeks 2 through 8. As osteoid is secreted, growth factors are released, which stimulate osteoclastic activity, leading to the remodeling phase of bone healing, which lasts from about week 8 throughout the life of the bone. Approximately 90% of the grafted site will be mature bone by 6 months.

The preferred situation with bone graft healing is to have regeneration of bone and not scar formation. There are several principles that must be adhered to in order for this to occur. First is an adequate blood supply. The blood supply for the grafted material initially comes from the adjacent native bone and the remaining soft tissues at the site. Early in the reparative phase of healing, there is vascularization of the grafted material. There also must be stabilization of the graft. Gross motion at the graft site will lead to fibrocartilage formation and to nonunion of the graft. Micromotion at the graft site cannot be avoided and may actually be beneficial to graft maturation, acting as a mechanical signal to stimulate graft healing.

SOFT TISSUE MANAGEMENT

Soft tissue management at the bone graft site is important to graft survival. An intact periosteum will provide a barrier from the oral cavity as well as a source for graft containment if primary closure of the site can be obtained. The periosteum is also a source of vascular supply for the graft.[4,5] With continuity defects and the use of cortical block grafts, primary closure over the graft site is essential. Exposure of the block graft will lead to loss of the entire graft. The use of particulate graft material is more forgiving. Exposure of the particulate material may not lead to loss of the entire graft. Gentle debridement of the exposed material and meticulous oral hygiene and wound care may allow for preservation of a portion of the grafted material. Some containment systems such as titanium mesh are forgiving, and with exposure, lead to minimal bone graft loss.[6,7]

Immediate bone grafting of extraction sites is often used in oral and maxillofacial surgery practices for the patient interested in implant restorations. Many methods for management of the soft tissue with these grafts have been proposed. For the best esthetic outcome, primary closure of these sites may not be ideal. One must consider graft containment also. Methods for containing the graft material and obtaining an excellent esthetic and functional outcome include primary closure, placement of a collagen plug over the graft material, nonvascularized connective tissue graft over the graft material, vascularized adjacent connective tissue transfer, and use of allogeneic, xenogenic, and synthetic membranes.[8–11]

TYPES OF BONE DEFECTS

Bony defects are classified in many ways (**Figs. 1** and **2**). The importance of the type of defect present is that it will dictate what type of grafting technique is used for reconstruction. The simplest classification is to describe the direction of bone loss. Horizontal bone loss indicates that there is loss of bone width. Vertical bone loss is loss of bone height. Vertical alveolar bone loss is more difficult to reconstruct than horizontal bone loss.

Another classification scheme is to define the defect based on the number of bony walls remaining at the site to be grafted. Total vertical bone loss is a single walled defect, and due to the limited amount of remaining native bone, it is the most challenging to reconstruct. A fresh extraction socket has five remaining walls (buccal, lingual, mesial, distal, and floor or apical bone) and

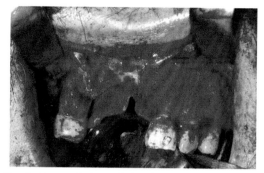

Fig. 1. Traumatic loss of alveolus. Demonstrates both horizontal and vertical bone loss.

provides much native bone and ease of graft containment.

GRAFT FUNCTION

Bone grafting materials affect new bone formation at the defect site in many ways. The material can induce bone formation through cellular signaling or through the transfer of osteocompetent cells, or it may simply provide a scaffolding and have a space maintaining function for the host to grow new bone. Graft materials therefore can be classified on their function and interaction with the host.

A graft that transfers osteocompetent cells that begin the bone forming process is called an osteogenic graft. The new bone at the site is formed from the cells transferred in the graft and not just from the osteocompetent cells at the defect site. The only osteogenic graft is an autogenous bone graft.

A graft that stimulates the host mesenchymal stem cells to differentiate and begin bone formation is called an osteoinductive graft. This process occurs through the transfer of proteins in the graft,

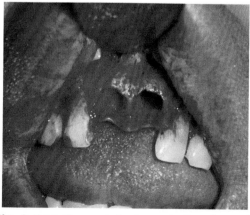

Fig. 2. Extraction sockets demonstrating five wall bony defects.

which begin a signaling cascade for the host to form bone.

A graft that simply provides scaffolding for the host to create new bone and has no biologic influence on the host is an osteoconductive graft. There are no proteins or cells present in the graft material to affect the host and influence bone formation.

Classification of Graft Types

Bone grafting materials can be subclassified many ways using a combination of their source of origin and mineral content (**Figs. 3** and **4**). The source can be subclassified further by species and by where in the bone the graft is taken.

Cortical bone is a graft taken from the outer compact bone of the graft source. It can be delivered in a particulate or block form by simple processing measures. Cancellous graft material is taken from the softer trabecular bone. It is usually found in a particulate form, but with proper processing it also can be offered as part of a block form.

Block bone grafts are typically cortical in nature. They hold their form very well and can be shaped and formed with many different types of instruments. Block bone can be from multiple sources. There are allografts, xenografts, and even synthetic block grafts available. Multiple autogenous intraoral and extraoral sites can be used to harvest block grafts including the mandibular ramus, the zygomatic buttress, the mental region of the mandible, the cranium, and the anterior and posterior iliac crests.

As discussed earlier, particulate grafts have the advantage of being able to withstand exposure to the oral cavity without total graft loss better than block grafts. Particulate grafts are available from

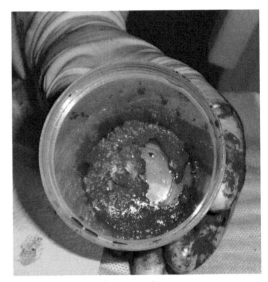

Fig. 4. Autogenous bone graft.

multiple biologic and synthetic sources. These grafts can be cortical, cancellous, or a cortical and cancellous mixture. Most manufacturers and processors offer the grafts with multiple particle sizes.

Another method of classifying grafts is based on their source (**Table 1**).[12] The gold standard in bone grafting materials is autogenous bone. This bone is harvested from the subject to which it is being grafted. There is no antigenic response to the grafted material and no chance of graft rejection. There are multiple sites for harvesting these grafts. Autogenous bone is the only source for transfer of viable osteoprogenitor cells and proteins. The disadvantage to autogenous grafts is the

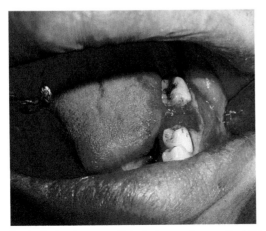

Fig. 3. Socket bone graft technique using particulate mixed (cortical and cancellous) allograft.

Table 1 Graft classification based on source	
Autograft	Taken from the host; The gold standard in bone grafting The only graft source that is osteogenic
Allograft	Graft taken from a genetically similar donor Cadaveric graft
Xenograft	Graft taken from a genetically dissimilar donor Most commonly bovine or porcine source
Synthetic graft	Graft not taken from a living donor No cellular or protein products in this graft

additional time and often additional surgical site required for harvesting the graft. Autogenous grafts provide all three functional properties of a graft material: osteogenesis, osteoinduction, and osteoconduction.

Another graft type is the allograft. This graft material also is known as a homologous graft, because it is taken from a genetically similar donor. The most common source of allograft is from cadaveric donors. These grafts are processed to reduce antigenicity, and through this process, all cellular material is killed. Therefore, there is no ability for transfer of osteocompetent cells with this graft type. Although never reported and very unlikely because of stringent donor selection and processing protocols, there is a chance for infectious disease transmission with allografts. Most patients, with proper counseling, will accept this risk easily. Allografts are available commercially in many forms including block grafts, particulate mineralized cortical, cancellous, mixed cortical/cancellous, and demineralized. The particulate grafts are also available with varying particle sizes. The grafts have the advantage of saving surgical time and no additional surgical harvest site. Allografts provide the graft functions of osteoinduction and osteoconduction.

Xenografts also are known as heterografts, because they are from genetically dissimilar, nonhuman sources. These grafts share many of the same advantages and disadvantages of the allografts. One difference is that the xenograft has the highest antigenic potential because of its being from a nonhuman source. These grafts also are processed to decrease the antigenicity, and there is a decreased chance for infectious disease transmission as well. Common sources for xenografts are bovine and porcine animals. Xenografts provide the graft functions of osteoinduction and osteoconduction.

Synthetic graft materials are also available. The ideal synthetic material is slowly resorbable and will maintain space for bone formation. These grafts are available in block and particulate forms. There is no cellular or protein material with these grafts. Their functional classification is only osteoconduction.

GRAFT CONTAINMENT AND FIXATION

In order for the graft to heal and allow for new bone formation, it must be contained at the site of the defect. Many different systems for graft containment are commercially available. The type of containment or fixation the surgeon chooses will be based upon location of the defect and the type of graft material used. For defects with adequate space maintenance of the surrounding tissue, the only containment required is an intact periosteum.

Particulate grafts require a containment system that keeps the graft material at the site, assists with maintaining space for bone regeneration, withstands exposure to the oral environment, prevents soft tissue ingrowth, and slowly resorbs or is easily removed (**Figs. 5** and **6**).[9] Common resorbable membranes are made from xenogenic collagen sources or cadaveric dermis. These membranes are slowly resorbable or are integrated into the adjacent soft tissue but have the disadvantage of poor space maintenance for the graft. They are best suited for use to prevent soft tissue ingrowth and with grafts that are not reliant on the membrane for structural support. Common nonresorbable containment systems include PTFE and titanium mesh. These are excellent sources for graft containment. and with titanium reinforced PTFE, there is excellent space maintenance with these materials. One major disadvantage of these is the difficulty encountered with their removal. Titanium mesh is excellent for space maintenance and with exposure to the oral cavity will still allow for graft healing.[7] Many synthetic resorbable mesh materials are available for graft containment. They are easily formed to the desired shape and are slowly resorbed. These materials do not tolerate intraoral exposure very well, and with

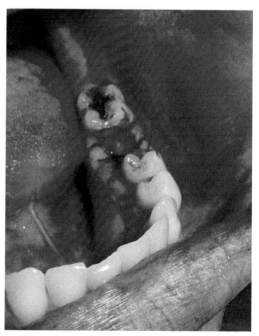

Fig. 5. Socket bone grafting technique demonstrating containment of the particulate bone graft material with a collagen plug and figure of eight suture.

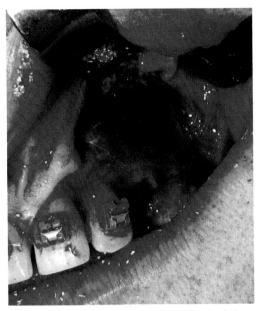

Fig. 6. Graft containment using a resorbable foil.

exposure can lead to total graft loss and multiple debridement procedures.

Block grafts require fixation of the graft at the site, prevention of gross motion, protection from the oral environment, and slow resorption or easy removal of the fixation. These goals can be accomplished with many commercially available systems. Continuity defects require the placement of a titanium reconstruction bar to maintain the proper space of the defect. This fixation device can be used for fixation of a block graft. For the small block graft used for alveolar reconstruction, miniplates and screw fixation work well. Positional and lag screw techniques may be used for fixation of the graft, and if properly placed, the screws can be removed easily with a small stab incision. Miniplates are excellent for graft fixation but require more extensive dissection for removal. Resorbable screws are also available for block graft fixation. The disadvantage with resorbable screws is the length of time for complete resorption and remaining material at the graft site at implant placement time.

SUMMARY

For many oral and maxillofacial surgeons, bone grafting is a daily procedure. This article was designed to review the principles of bone healing and bone grafting. There are many different ways to reach the same goal when bone grafting procedures are performed. With all of the available methods and materials, a clear understanding of these basic principles will assist in the selection of a technique for each individual patient.

REFERENCES

1. Olsen B, Reginato A, Wang W. Bone development. Annu Rev Cell Dev Biol 2000;16:191–220.
2. Chen JH, Liu C, You L, et al. Boning up on Wolff's law: mechanical regulation of the cells that make and maintain bone. J Biomech 2009;43:108–18.
3. Marx R. Bone and bone graft healing. Oral Maxillofac Surg Clin North Am 2007;19:455–66.
4. Takushima A, Kitano Y, Harii K. Osteogenic potential of cultured periosteal cells in a distracted bone gap in rabbits. J Surg Res 1998;78:68–77.
5. Simpson A. The blood supply of the periosteum. J Anat 1985;140:697–704.
6. Gutta R, Baker R, Bartolucci A, et al. Barrier membranes used for ridge augmentation: is there an optimal pore size? J Oral Maxillofac Surg 2009; 67:1218–25.
7. Louis P, Gutta R, Said-Al-Naief N, et al. Reconstruction of the maxilla and mandible with particulate bone graft and titanium mesh for implant placement. J Oral Maxillofac Surg 2008;66:235–45.
8. Jung R, Siegenthaler D, Hammerle C. Postextraction tissue management: a soft tissue punch technique. Int J Periodontics Restorative Dent 2004;24:545–53.
9. Block M. Treatment of the single tooth extraction site. Oral Maxillofac Surg Clin North Am 2004;16:41–63.
10. Wang H, Kiyonobu K, Neiva RF, et al. Socket augmentation: rationale and technique. Implant Dent 2004;13:286–93.
11. Wang H, Tsao Y. Mineralized bone allograft-plug socket augmentation: rationale and technique. Implant Dent 2007;16:33–7.
12. Kao S, Scott D. A review of bone substitutes. Oral Maxillofac Surg Clin North Am 2007;19:513–21.

Bone Graft Harvesting From Distant Sites: Concepts and Techniques

Kenneth J. Zouhary, DDS, MD[a,b,*]

KEYWORDS

- Graft • Harvest • Iliac • Tibial • Cranial • Calvarial

BACKGROUND

Reconstruction of the moderately to severely resorbed maxillary and mandibular alveolar bone in preparation for endosseous dental implant placement can be one of the most challenging tasks presenting to the oral and maxillofacial surgeon. Bell[1] summarized the aim of bone grafting over 40 years ago "to place a readily vascularizable osteogenic organic structure in intimate contact with a vascular osteogenic cancellous host bed" while adhering to "sound orthopedic principles." A number of autogenous, allogeneic, xenogeneic, and alloplastic grafts have been employed alone or in various combinations to meet this challenge.

The ideal bone graft material for implant reconstruction should have the following characteristics. The graft material should have the structural integrity to maintain space during bone ingrowth, graft consolidation and maturation, and implant osseointegration. It should be able to promote cells at the recipient site to form bone within the graft. The graft material should be able to be resorbed, remodeled, and replaced as the viable native bone. The resultant augmented alveolus should be stable over time after implant restoration and functional loading. The material should have ease of harvest (if autogenous) and placement to minimize procedure length, thus maximizing potential for graft success while minimizing patient morbidity. The graft should have a repeatable and predictable outcome.[2]

Although there is no ideal bone graft, autogenous bone remains the gold standard for alveolar reconstruction as it possesses the three classic qualities of the ideal graft, including osteoinduction, osteoconduction, and osteogenesis. Osteoconduction is the passive ingrowth of vascular tissue and mesenchymal stem cells into the scaffold structure presented by the graft material. Osteoinduction is a two-stage process, which includes cell recruitment and cell differentiation. The first stage of osteoinduction involves the active recruitment of undifferentiated mesenchymal stem cells to the graft site by bone morphogenic proteins present within the graft material. The second stage involves triggering of the stem cells to differentiate into osteoblasts. Osteogenesis refers to the transfer of osteoprogenitor cells already present within the graft. Inherent to the concept of osteogenesis is the cells' ability to survive the transplant, proliferate at the recipient site, and differentiate into osteoblasts. Osteoconduction is a property that most graft materials possess. Many bone graft materials also contain various amounts of osteoinductive potential. This osteoinductivity is often unpredictable and inconsistent even within the same grafting material. Osteogenesis, however, is unique to autogenous bone grafts and is arguably the most important quality of the three.

a Department of Oral and Maxillofacial Surgery, Birmingham VA Medical Center, 700 19th Street South, Birmingham, AL 35233, USA
b Department of Oral and Maxillofacial Surgery, University of Alabama at Birmingham, 2000 6th Avenue South, Birmingham, AL 35233,USA
* Department of Oral and Maxillofacial Surgery, Birmingham VA Medical Center, 700 19th Street South, Birmingham, AL 35233.
E-mail address: kzouhary@uab.edu

Oral Maxillofacial Surg Clin N Am 22 (2010) 301–316
doi:10.1016/j.coms.2010.04.007
1042-3699/10/$ – see front matter. Published by Elsevier Inc.

When selecting the appropriate bone graft source, there are multiple factors that one must consider with regards to the recipient site, the donor site, and the patient. One must first consider the size of the defect to be restored to help determine the quantity of bone graft required. One must also decide what type of defect is to be restored to determine the quality of graft required: cortical versus cancellous. Operative time and donor site morbidity are major factors to be considered and help to guide the choice of graft material. Only after careful consideration of these factors in light of the patient's comorbidities and expectations will one be able to select the appropriate harvest site for each particular patient and application.

Much of what is known about the behavior of various autogenous bone grafts to the dental alveolus comes from past experience with congenital alveolar cleft defects. Early animal studies showed that membranous bone grafts maintained volume better than endochondral bone grafts when used as a corticocancellous onlay graft. This led to a consensus that membranous bone grafts were superior to endochondral grafts based on their embryologic origin. Thus cranial bone and mandibular bone were often preferred for onlay grafting in craniofacial applications. Ozaki and Buchman[3] hypothesized that membranous bone resorbed less over time compared with endochondral bone because of its microarchitectural features (relative cortical and cancellous composition) rather than its embryologic superiority. They found no statistical difference in rate of resorption between two cortical onlay grafts of different embryologic origin when the cortical and cancellous components were separated. Rosenthal and Buchman[4] proceeded to examine the behavior of embryologically diverse bone grafts in inlay grafts as opposed to onlay grafts. They created four critical size defects in rabbit crania and grafted each with either membranous cortical, endochondral cortical, endochondral cancellous, or a control consisting of no bone graft at all. They found that all three grafted sites increased in bone volume compared with the control. Interestingly, they found that the endochondral cancellous bone volume increased the most. They concluded that the ratio of cortical to cancellous graft was far more influential in graft performance than embryologic origin. They also concluded that inlay grafts behave differently than onlay grafts, thus the selection of donor site must fit the type of defect to be corrected.

Autogenous bone can be harvested from either intraoral or extraoral (distant) sites. Intraoral harvest sites include, but are not limited to, the mandibular symphysis, external oblique ridge,

ramus, retromolar pad, alveolus, tori, tuberosity, and zygomatic buttress. Intraoral bone grafts are not typically limited by their quality but rather by their quantity. When larger alveolar augmentations and jaw reconstructions are undertaken, extraoral harvest sites can be exploited for increased amounts of cortical and cancellous bone.

Extraoral harvest sites typically used in jaw reconstruction include the iliac crest, the proximal tibia, the calvarium, and the rib. Although historically popular for preprosthetic ridge augmentation, rib grafts have been largely abandoned as a graft source for alveolar reconstruction due to the inferior bone quality and severe resorption observed under the compressive forces of the masticatory apparatus. More recently, osseous free flaps have been employed in alveolar reconstruction in combination with endosseous implants.[5] These osseous flaps are often used in conjunction with oncologic postablative or post-traumatic reconstruction and fall outside of the scope of this article.

The volume of bone available for harvest from extraoral sites is quite variable depending on patient factors such as size, age, and gender. The average volumes reported in the literature are even further confounded by the inconsistent degree of graft compression. Whereas the calvarium contains large amounts of cortical bone and the tibia houses large amounts of cancellous bone, the iliac crest is a reservoir of large amounts of both cortical and cancellous bone. The anterior iliac crest can yield 50 cc of particulate bone and uncompressed marrow or a corticocancellous block of 5 × 3 cm. The posterior iliac crest can produce 100 to 125 cc of corticocancellous bone or a 5 × 5 cm block. 25 to 40 cc of non-compressed cancellous bone can be harvested from the proximal tibia. The calvarium provides abundant cortical bone from the outer cortex and variable amounts of cancellous bone from the diploic space (**Table 1**).

ANTERIOR ILIAC CREST BONE GRAFT

The anterior iliac crest bone graft (AICBG) is advantageous as it can provide up to 50 cc of corticocancellous graft of excellent quality. It allows for two surgical teams with simultaneous graft harvest and recipient site preparation. The major disadvantages of this harvest site are risk of sensory nerve injury and gait instability.

The relevant anatomy includes the bony landmarks of the anterior superior iliac spine (ASIS) and the iliac tubercle, which lies approximately 6 cm posterior to the ASIS. In a cadaveric study by Ebraheim and colleagues,[6] the thickest portion of

Table 1
Typical noncompressed graft volumes available for harvest

	Noncompressed Cortico-Cancellous	Cortical Block
Tibia	25–40 cc	1 × 2 cm
Anterior Ilium	50 cc	3 × 5 cm
Posterior Ilium	100–125 cc	5 × 5 cm
Calvarium	variable, minimal	abundant

the ilium was 16.9 ± 2.3 mm at the iliac tubercle, which was 45% thicker than at a point 3 cm posterior to the anterior superior iliac spine. The thickest region of the crest extended 54.0 ± 10.2 mm posteriorly from a point 3 cm posterior to the anterior superior iliac spine. The relevant muscular anatomy includes the external oblique, tensor fascia lata, gluteus medius, and iliacus. Blood supply to the iliac crest comes from the deep circumflex iliac artery and the most common source of significant bleeding during harvest comes from a branch of the internal iliac artery, namely the superior gluteal artery. Sensory nerves at risk of injury include the lateral cutaneous branch of the subcostal nerve, the lateral cutaneous branch of the iliohypogastric nerve, and the lateral femoral cutaneous nerve. There is some conflicting data as to the most commonly injured nerve during graft harvest with each of the three sensory nerves being cited by different authors (**Fig. 1**).[7–9] Chou and colleagues[9] demonstrated the subcostal nerve to be at particular risk during this dissection. Bilateral dissections were performed on 10 cadavers and the nerves were traced back to their spinal origins. The subcostal nerve was found to be 6 to 11 cm posterior to the ASIS with a mean distance of 9 cm. A separate study of 54 cadaveric specimens showed an anomalous course of the lateral femoral cutaneous nerve in 4% of the dissections with the nerve crossing 2 to 3 cm posterior to the ASIS, placing it at considerable risk during dissection.[10] A third cadaveric study found just one lateral branch of the lateral femoral cutaneous nerve out of 34 dissections (2.9%) crossing at a distance less than 5 mm posterior to the ASIS.[11] It is important to avoid the lateral femoral cutaneous nerve as direct trauma or stretch injury can result in the very painful neuropathy meralgia paresthetica.

The incision to the anterior iliac crest is designed with the overlying skin retracted medially to prevent the surgical scar from lying directly over the crest of the ridge and causing irritation from clothing resting on the crest of the ridge (**Fig. 2**). A 4 to 6 cm incision is performed starting 2 cm posterior to the ASIS to avoid the lateral femoral cutaneous nerve and extending posteriorly toward the tubercle. Dissection is carried through skin and subcutaneous tissue down to the muscles. The dissection continues through the aponeurosis between the external oblique and tensor fascia lata muscles. The periosteum is sharply elevated off the crest of the ridge and the Iliacus muscle is retracted medially in a subperiosteal plane. A cortical block graft can then be harvested from the medial aspect of the crest and cancellous bone can then be harvested using bone curettes. After bone graft harvest, hemostasis is achieved using cautery, bone wax, microfibrillar collagen, or Gelfoam. Drain placement is optional but not necessary. Closure is achieved with multilayered closure of the periosteum, muscular aponeurosis, and skin.

Alternative graft harvest techniques have been used successfully such as trephine, bicortical, and tricortical grafts, including the medial and lateral cortices as well as the crest of the ridge. In a randomized prospective study, Tayapongsak and colleagues[12] found no significant difference between a medial and lateral approach with regards to postoperative morbidity. Falkensammer and colleagues[13] described a technique for bicortical graft without disruption of the iliac crest by removing a window of bicortical bone below the crest from a lateral approach. Grillon and colleagues[14] described a graft modification by raising a laterally based osteoperiosteal flap from the crest of the ilium and removing a medial corticocancellous bone block; thus maintaining the normal crest anatomy and potentially decreasing postoperative morbidity. When a full thickness tricortical graft is taken, immediate reconstruction of the iliac crest has been shown to decrease postoperative pain and cosmetic deformity.[15,16] When only cancellous bone is required, one of four classic harvest techniques can be used.[8] The clamshell involves cortical expansion. The trap door employs a medial or lateral pedicle of the crestal cortex. The Tschopp technique uses a single oblique osteotomy and the Tessier technique uses both medial and lateral oblique osteotomies.

Complications associated with the AICBG are reported to range between 1% and 25% and include hematoma, seroma, nerve injury, cosmetic deformity, pelvic instability, abdominal hernia, ileus, perforation, infection, persistent pain, and iliac crest fracture (**Box 1**). De Riu and colleagues[17] reported a massive iliac abscess that presented 4

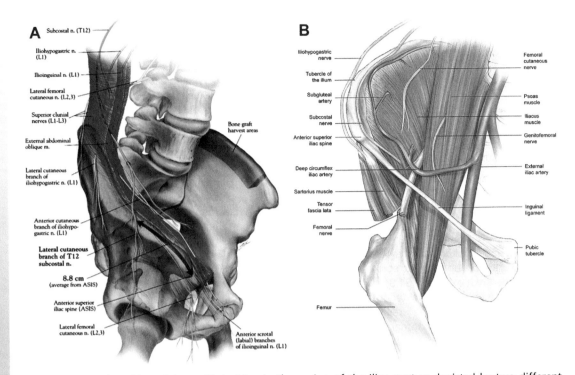

Fig. 1. Nerves vulnerable to injury with incision in the region of the iliac crest as depicted by two different authors. (*A*) The lateral branch of the subcostal nerve is shown to be especially vulnerable to injury where the grafts are harvested from the anterior crest. M, muscle; n, nerve. (*From* Chou D, Storm PB, Campbell JN. Vulnerability of the subcostal nerve to injury during bone graft harvesting from the iliac crest. J Neurosurg 2004;1:87–9; with permission.) (*B*) Relationship of the iliohypogastric nerve to the iliac tubercle, placing it at considerable risk during bone harvest from the iliac crest. (*From* Kademani D, Keller E. Iliac crest grafting for mandibular reconstruction. Atlas Oral Maxillofac Surg Clin North Am 2006;14:161–70; with permission.)

years after graft harvest. It is recommended to use a reciprocating saw and to stay at least 3 cm posterior to the ASIS to prevent fracture of the iliac crest or spine.[18] When fracture is encountered, it is typically treated with conservative measures such as bed rest or weight bearing as tolerated on the affected side.

POSTERIOR ILIAC CREST BONE GRAFT

The posterior iliac crest bone graft (PICBG) for maxillofacial reconstruction was first described in 1980 by Bloomquist and Feldman.[19] It is advantageous over the anterior approach as it contains a considerable amount of available bone graft, and it has a lower incidence of postoperative pain and gait disturbance. Disadvantages of the posterior approach include increased operative time with patient repositioning and increased anesthetic risks associated with prone positioning. Another disadvantage is that this approach does not allow for simultaneous harvest with two surgical teams.

The majority of the bone available for harvest lies beneath the insertion of the gluteus maximus on the 3 × 4 cm triangular tubercle adjacent to the sacroiliac joint. The average maximum thickness of the bone in this region is 17.1 mm.[20] The gluteus medius muscle inserts anterior to the gluteus maximus. The dissection is performed between the superior cluneal (L1-L3) and middle cluneal (S1-S3) cutaneous nerves. The sciatic notch lies approximately 10 to 12 cm inferior to the iliac crest. The medial cortex of the iliac bone is lined by the iliacus muscle. Perforating vessels off the deep circumflex iliac artery provide blood supply to the bone. A terminal branch of the deep circumflex iliac artery, the subgluteal artery, courses through the sciatic notch and ramifies along the ilium in the area of the triangular tubercle. In a cadaveric study, Xu and colleagues[20] analyzed bony features of the posterior ilium and relevant vital structures. The average distance from the PSIS to the superior cluneal nerves was 68.8 mm with a range of 64–78 mm. The average distance from the iliac crest to the superior gluteal vessels was 102.3 mm with a range of 92 to 114 mm.

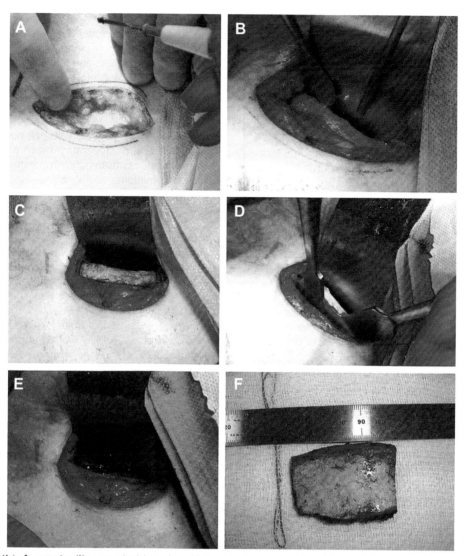

Fig. 2. (*A*) Left anterior iliac crest incision placed lateral to the crest of the ridge and 2 cm posterior to ASIS. Incision carried down through the aponeurosis between the tensor fascia lata laterally and the external oblique muscle medially. (*B*) Exposure of the bony crest of the ridge with subperiosteal reflection of the iliacus muscle using a periosteal elevator followed by a malleable retractor. (*C*) Bony osteotomies made with reciprocating saw 3 cm posterior to ASIS and extending 5 cm posteriorly (ASIS marked with horizontal surgical marking pen). (*D*) Corticocancellous block graft gently separated from lateral cortex using paired osteotomes. (*E*) Donor site after removal of block graft demonstrating remaining cancellous bone available for harvest with bone curettes. (*F*) Corticocancellous block graft harvested approximately 5 × 3 cm.

Surgical approach to the posterior iliac crest begins with the patient positioned prone with 210° reverse hip flexion. A 6 to 10 cm curvilinear incision is made over the triangular tubercle, staying a minimum of 3 cm from the midline (**Fig. 3**). Dissection is carried through the skin, subcutaneous tissue, thoracodorsal fascia, and periosteum. The thoracodorsal fascia can be identified as a thick white fascial layer and it is the caudal extension of the latissimus dorsi. The

gluteus maximus is sharply elevated off the tubercle. Only a small portion of the gluteus medius muscle is elevated in a subperiosteal plane. A 5 × 5 cm lateral cortical block graft can be harvested extending along the crest of the ridge of the triangular tubercle. Cancellous bone can then be harvested with bone gouges and bone curettes. Hemostasis is achieved with cautery, bone wax, microfibrillar collagen, or Gelfoam. Multilayered closure is achieved with closure of the periosteum

Box 1
Complications associated with anterior iliac crest bone graft harvest

Hematoma

Seroma

Paresthesia

Cosmetic deformity

Pelvic instability

Abdominal hernia

Ileus

Infection

Persistent pain

Fracture

Potential complications of the posterior iliac crest bone harvest include, but are not limited to, compartment syndrome from subgluteal artery bleeding, ureteral injury, abdominal hernia, or cluneal nerve injury **Box 2**. In a series of 839 harvests over 25 years, Marx[21] reported seroma to be the most common postoperative complication with an incidence of 3.6%. He also reported six hematomas (0.7%), four patients with gait disturbance (0.5%), and one postoperative bleed (0.1%). He reported no symptomatic paresthesias or neuroma formations.

Several prospective studies looking at the rate of persistent pain and morbidity from PICBG harvest have come from the orthopedic literature. These prospective studies showed persistent pain and morbidity from iliac crest bone graft harvest for spinal fusion to be higher than previously reported. At 1 year postoperative, 16.5% of patients reported more severe pain from the harvest site than the primary surgical site and 29.1% reported numbness. With respect to functional limitations resulting from harvest site pain, 15.1% reported some difficulty walking, 5.2% with work activity, 12.9% with

and gluteus maximus followed by the thoracodorsal fascia, subcutaneous tissue, and skin. A drain is typically placed and left to bulb suction. The site is then covered with microfoam tape and the patient is repositioned to the supine position for oral reconstruction.

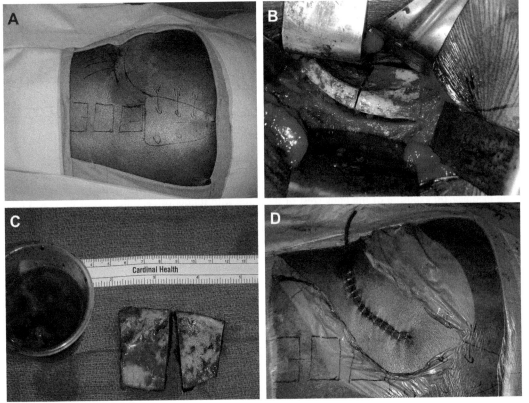

Fig. 3. (*A*) Right-sided posterior iliac crest bone harvest depicting the location of the superior and middle cluneal nerves to the palpable bony landmarks. (*B*) Corticotomies along the crest of the ridge and the lateral cortices with gluteus maximus reflected. (*C*) Corticocancellous blocks and cancellous bone harvested from the posterior hip. (*D*) Closure of the incision with suction bulb drain in place laterally.

<table>
<tr><td>

Box 2
Complications associated with posterior iliac crest bone graft harvest

Bleeding

Ureteral injury

Abdominal hernia

Paresthesia

Seroma

Hematoma

Gait disturbance

Infection

Scarring

</td></tr>
</table>

recreation, 14.1% with household chores, 7.6% with sexual activity, and 5.9% irritation from clothing.[22] In a separate study, at 3.5 years mean follow-up, 24% of patients reported harvest site numbness, and 13% reported the numbness as bothersome. Harvest site pain resulted in functional limitations with walking in 16% of patients, 10% with work activity, 18% with recreation, 19% with household chores, 16% with sexual activity, and irritation from clothing with 9%. These rates of functional limitation are much higher than previously reported and may be due to the increased sensitivity of the prospective study design or targeted investigation of these specific symptoms. Validity of these findings is limited by patient ability to discriminate harvest site pain from postsurgical or chronic back pain.[23]

AICBG VERSUS PICBG

One advantage of the anterior approach is that a bicortical or tricortical graft can be harvested from the anterior ilium. The posterior harvest is limited to the lateral cortex and the crest of the ridge since the medial aspect of the ilium contributes to the sacroiliac joint. The posterior ilium contains significantly more cancellous bone than the anterior ilium. This is partly due to increased surface area of the posterior ilium, but it is also due to the greater medial-lateral depth of the posterior iliac marrow space. A comparative anatomic study of the anterior and posterior iliac crests showed the surgically accessible marrow space to be 15.75 mL for the anterior and 39.24 mL for the posterior ilium with a ratio of compressed cancellous bone from the posterior to anterior ilium of 2.4:1.[24] Marx and Morales[25] compared the morbidity of the AICBG with the PICBG in a randomized prospective study in 100 consecutive patients with continuity defects of 6

cm or greater, thus requiring at least 60 cc cancellous bone. They found the posterior approach to have decreased morbidity in all parameters measured including pain, ambulation, seroma, and blood loss (**Table 2**).

In a prospective nonrandomized study of 118 patients, Kessler and colleagues[26] compared the volume of bone harvested, the operating time, and the postoperative morbidity between the AICBG (81 cases) and the PICBG (46 cases). The mean volume of bone harvested from the anterior crest was 9 cc (range 5–2) and from the posterior crest 25.5 cc (range 17–29). The mean operating time for the anterior approach was 35 minutes (range 22–48). The mean operating time for the posterior approach was 40 minutes (range 32–55). This did not include the additional time required for patient repositioning and redraping with a mean time of 20 minutes (range 14–27). The posterior approach caused less morbidity particularly with respect to the statistically significant decrease in pain and gait disturbance (**Table 3**).

Nkenke and colleagues[27] showed gait disturbance and pain scores to be higher in the AICBG early on as compared with the PICBG, but no difference at 1 month postoperative. An extensive review of the literature focusing on anterior and posterior iliac fractures after graft harvest was reported by Nocini and colleagues[28] in 2003. Of the 35 cases reported in the literature at that time, 24 fractures were associated with harvesting from the anterior crest and 12 were due to posterior crest harvest. Four out of 24 anterior fractures required further surgical treatment (16.6%). Eight of the 12 posterior fractures required one or more additional surgical procedures (66.6%). Although painful, fractures of the anterior iliac crest remain stable and heal spontaneously in most cases without further complication. On the contrary, fractures of the posterior iliac crest due to graft harvest often require further surgical intervention and functional disability.

TIBIAL BONE GRAFT

Bone graft harvest from the proximal tibia has been well established as a source of cancellous bone with minimal morbidity.[29] Catone and colleagues[30] first described the use of this site in reconstruction of the maxilla and maxilla. Advantages to the proximal tibia as a donor site include a low complication rate, a large amount of cancellous bone available, it is a technically simple and quick procedure, it allows for simultaneous harvest and recipient site preparation, and it can decrease costs to the patient as it can be

Table 2
Donor site morbidity from anterior and posterior iliac crest graft harvest

	Anterior Approach n = 50	Posterior Approach n = 50	P Value
Mean first day of ambulation	3.6 days	1.7 days	.005
Seroma	12% (6/50)	2% (1/50)	.005
Hematoma	6% (3/50)	0% (0/50)	.050
Fracture	2% (1/50)	0% (0.50)	.010
Pain level, day 1	7.2/10	3.1/10	.005
Pain level, day 10	4.4/10	0.3/10	.005
Limp, day 10	42% (21/50)	6% (3/50)	.005
Limp, day 60	15% (8/50)	0% (0.50)	.005

Data from Marx RE, Morales MJ. Morbidity from bone harvest in major jaw reconstruction: a randomized trial comparing the lateral anterior and posterior approaches to the ilium. J Oral Maxillofac Surg 1988;48:196–203.

performed as an outpatient or in office procedure. Reported disadvantages include the limited amount of cortical bone available for harvest, variable amount of cancellous bone, and the quality of the cancellous bone.

Many of the reports of the volume of cancellous bone available for harvest are based on retrospective review of cases performed. The amount of bone harvested in these cases may be based on the amount of bone required for reconstruction rather than the amount of bone available. Also, the literature is inconsistent with regards to reporting of compressed versus noncompressed bone. To determine the amount of bone available for harvest Wang and colleagues[31] performed a volumetric analysis of the proximal tibia using a three-dimensional imaging reconstruction of 18 adult CT scans. They reported an average of 77 cm^2 of cancellous bone available for harvest in the proximal tibia. This is two to three times the accepted average. Tibial bone has a higher composition of fat as compared with iliac cancellous grafts. The gross discrepancy between the results of this imaging study and clinical studies is due not only to incomplete harvest of the available bone, but also due to compression of the cancellous bone during harvest and before reporting. It is important to compress the cancellous bone to lyse and extrude the fat cells, concentrate the osteogenic progenitor cells, and to assist in more consistent reporting of volume of bone harvested. The easiest way to compress the harvested bone is in a 10 cc syringe (**Fig. 4**G).

There are very few studies comparing tibial bone and iliac crest as sources for bone grafts. The perception that the quality of cancellous bone from the tibia is of inferior quality as compared with the iliac crest is based mostly on anecdotal

Table 3
Complications after harvesting from the anterior and posterior iliac crest

Complication	Anterior (*n* = 81)	Posterior (*n* = 46)	Total (*n* = 127)	P Value
Seroma	1 (1%)	3 (6%)	4 (3%)	—
Hematoma	7 (9%)	2 (4%)	9 (7%)	—
Infection	1 (1%)	0	1 (1%)	—
Hyperesthesia	1 (1%)	0	1 (1%)	—
Total	10 (12%)	5 (11%)	15 (12%)	—
Pain	57 (70%)	15 (33%)	72 (57%)	<.001
Irregularities of gait				
After 2 weeks	26 (32%)	3 (6%)	29 (23%)	.002
After 4 weeks	8 (10%)	1 (2%)	9 (7%)	—

Data from Kessler P, Thorwarth M, Bloch-Birkholz A, et al. Harvesting of bone from the iliac crest: comparison of the anterior and posterior sites. Br J Oral Maxillofac Surg 2005;43:51–6.

reports of the appearance of the bone at the time of harvest. This perception was challenged by a prospective study of 40 patients undergoing secondary bone grafting in alveolar clefts. This study showed similar optical bone densities in tibial and iliac crest bone grafts over the first 3 postoperative months. Another significant finding in this study was the shorter hospital stay for the patients in the tibial bone graft group.[32]

The classic approach to the cancellous bone present in the proximal tibial metaphysis is the lateral approach.[33] The lateral approach is centered over Gerdy's tubercle located between the tibial tuberosity and the fibular head (**Fig. 4**). There are no vital structures overlying Gerdy's tubercle making this a safe and effective approach. Sensory innervation in this area is supplied by cutaneous branches of the lateral sural nerve. The anterior tibialis muscle lies inferior to Gerdy's tubercle along with branches of the inferior genicular artery and the recurrent anterior tibial artery. Gerdy's tubercle is easily palpated in most patients and a 3 to 4 cm incision is made directly over Gerdy's tubercle. Dissection is carried through the skin, subcutaneous fat, iliotibial tract, and the periosteum. This tends to be a very dry dissection and tourniquet is not necessary. A 1 to 2 cm cortical window is then outlined with a fissure bur. An oval window is recommended as it produces less stress and reduces the risk of postoperative fracture. Bone curettes are then used to first harvest the cancellous bone across the plateau and finally down the shaft. Harvesting the shaft last rather than first prevents the more proximal bone from falling down the shaft delaying and complicating its removal. Caution must be used in harvesting bone superiorly to avoid entering the knee joint. If bleeding is encountered in this harvest, it is usually from cortical perforator vessels. A gelatin sponge or microfibrillar collagen can be placed in the bony cavity but is rarely needed. Layered closure includes the periosteum and iliotibial tract as one layer, followed by the skin. An Ace wrap is placed and the patient is permitted to ambulate that same day with weight bearing as tolerated. Rarely, a cane will be necessary to reduce fall risk, and patients are to avoid vigorous exercise for 6 weeks.

Alternate approaches to the tibial bone graft harvest include the medial approach (**Fig. 5**). Herford and colleagues[34] performed a study on 20 cadavers comparing the medial and lateral approaches. They found no statistical difference in the mean volume of bone harvested from either approach. They reported the thickness of the cortex medially and laterally to be 1.4 mm and 1.5 mm respectively. The incision for the medial approach is centered over a point 15 mm medial to the tibial parallel line and 15 mm superior to the tibial perpendicular line. This may be quite arbitrary as the tibial perpendicular line is based on accurate determination of the location of the center of the tibial tuberosity. This can be difficult to determine in larger individuals where the tuberosity may not be prominent. The relevant anatomy involves the pes ansernius which is the attachment of the sartorius, gracillus, and semitendinosus muscles. The pes is reported to be 4.85 mm inferior to the tibial perpendicular line. The medial approach is potentially advantageous as it is distant from any vital anatomic structures. In comparison the lateral approach is closer to vital structures such as the articular surface, the anterior tibialis muscle, and the anterior tibial vessels, and is located within the anterior compartment. Herford and colleagues[34] report that when using the medial approach the bone is closer to the skin, but this is debatable as Gerdy's tubercle is a palpable bony landmark close to the skin. In comparison, the medial approach incision is based on measurements from the tibial tuberosity which is often not as palpable as Gerdy's tubercle, making the dissection less predictable.

When lesser quantities of bone are required, bone trephination can be used for cancellous harvest with potentially less morbidity.[35–39] Although up to 40 mL of cancellous bone has been reported to be harvested with a trephine.[37] A major advantage of the tibial bone graft is that it is well tolerated in the outpatient clinic with intravenous conscious sedation.[39,40] It has also been described using only local anesthesia with good patient acceptance.[35,41]

Although tibial bone graft harvesting is a relatively simple and safe procedure, it is not without potential complication **Box 3**. Reported complications include prolonged pain, gait disturbance, wound dehiscence, infection, unaesthetic scarring, hematoma, seroma, paresthesia, fracture, and violation of the joint space. A recent meta-analysis by Schmidt and Townsend[42] found just 63 major and minor complications out of a collective group of 1,137 patients (5.5%). O'Keeffe and colleagues[29] reported a donor site complication rate of 1.3% in 230 harvests. Alt and colleagues[43] reported a complication rate of 1.9% with one postoperative hematoma and no major complications. Kushner[33] reported a 1.4% complication rate in a series of 141 patients including one wound dehiscence and one superficial infection. One case of early postoperative osteomyelitis requiring further surgical intervention and long term antimicrobials has been reported.[42] In a retrospective review of 75 patients undergoing

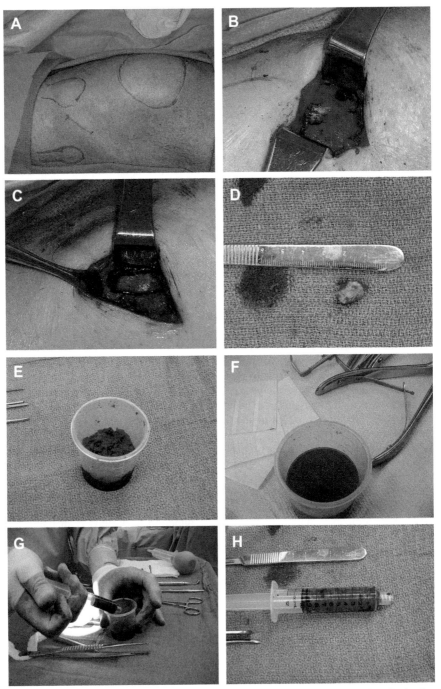

Fig. 4. (A) Bony landmarks for lateral approach to the left tibia highlighting the patella, tibial tuberosity, proximal fibula, and oblique incision overlying Gerdy's tubercle. (B) Exposure of Gerdy's tubercle. (C) Cortical osteotomy overlying Gerdy's tubercle. (D) Corticocancellous block harvest. (E) Cancellous bone harvest. (F) Fat droplets demonstrating fatty component of tibial bone. (G) Compression of cancellous bone. (H) Compressed tibial cancellous graft.

tibial bone graft for alveolar cleft bone grafting, Hughes and colleagues[44] reported two cases (2.7%) of proximal tibia fracture. Thor and colleagues[45] reported one case of tibial fracture secondary to graft requiring open reduction and internal fixation. A biomechanical study on human cadaveric tibia quantified the effect of various graft harvest defect sizes and locations

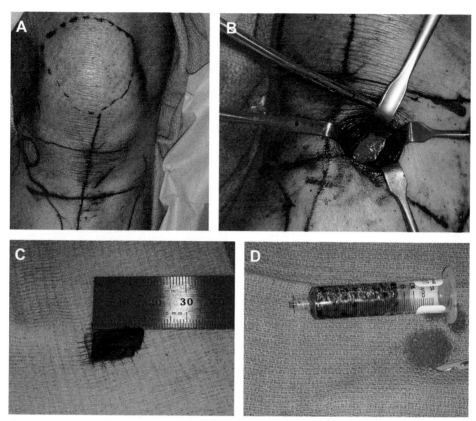

Fig. 5. (*A*) Medial approach for a right tibial bone harvest based on vertical and horizontal position of the tibial tuberosity (circle overlying Gerdy's tubercle laterally). (*B*) Cortical osteotomy demonstrating thickness of tissue overlying the medial approach as compared with the lateral approach. (*C*) Corticocancellous block harvested from tibia. (*D*) Compressed cancellous tibial bone.

on the deformation of the tibial plateau under load. Deformation of the plateau increased with both increased diameter of the defect and decreased distance between the defect and the plateau.[46]

Box 3
Complications associated with tibial bone graft harvest

Prolonged pain

Gait disturbance

Wound dehiscience

Infection

Scarring

Hematoma

Seroma

Paresthesia

Fracture

Violation of the joint space

A prospective study compared trephined bone grafts of the tibial shaft and iliac crest. There were no significant differences between the two groups with respect to objective assessment of postoperative pain or functional impairment, but the tibial trephine procedure was easier, quicker, and caused less blood loss. Subjective scores for pain and difficulty in ambulating were much lower for tibial bone grafts than for iliac crest bone grafts.[47]

CALVARIAL BONE GRAFT

Calvarial bone has been widely used in cranial reconstruction. Tessier's[48] landmark article in 1982 first described the use of autogenous calvarial bone grafts for facial reconstruction. The dense cortical nature of cranial bone makes it ideal as an onlay material as it has been shown to have rapid revascularization and decreased resorption as compared with corticocancellous onlay grafts. Ease of harvest, close proximity to the surgical site, minimal postoperative bony and soft tissue deformity, and quantity of bone available make this a good selection when moderate-to-large amounts of cortical bone graft are desired. Potential disadvantages of the calvarial bone graft include risk of dural tear, postoperative contour deformity, scarring, minimal cancellous bone available for harvest, and the close proximity to the recipient site which precludes the use of two surgical teams.[49] There are multiple surgical techniques described in harvesting the cranial bone,

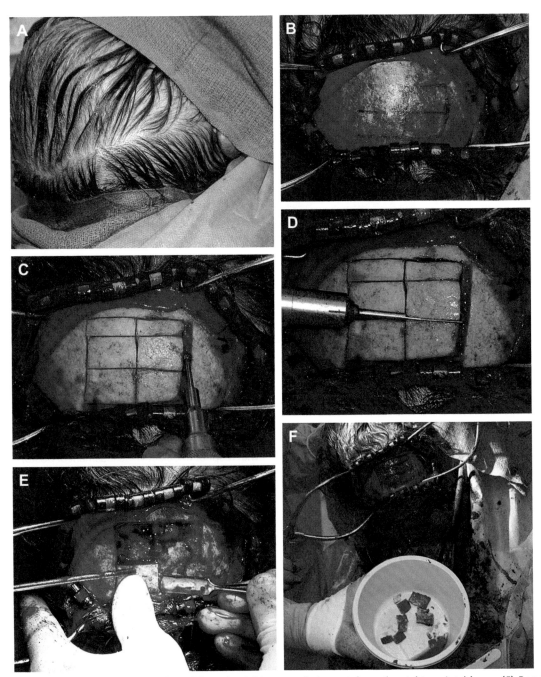

Fig. 6. (*A*) Patient prepped and draped for calvarial bone graft harvest from the right parietal bone. (*B*) Bone harvest exposure and surgical marking of proposed osteotomies with medial extent of osteotomy at least 2 cm from the midline to avoid the sagittal sinus. (*C*) Waste strip designed with round bur clearly showing the thickness of the outer cortical plate. (*D*) Corticotomies through the outer cortical plate with a reciprocating saw to 3 mm depth or the height of the saw blade tip. (*E*) Cortical blocks separated from inner table with osteotomes and mallet. (*F*) Harvested cortical block grafts and donor site before scalp closure.

although most involve the parietal bone because of its relative thickness and safety in harvest.

The local anatomy for the calvarial bone graft harvest is very straightforward. Typically the parietal bone is the preferred site as it has the maximal bone thickness and is located within the hair-bearing region of the scalp. Multiple studies have looked at the thickness of the skull, but the most comprehensive study to date measured 40 points on 281 dried skulls from the Cleveland Museum of Natural History. The average skull thickness was 6.3 mm ranging from 5.3 to 7.5 mm with a pattern of greatest thickness toward the posterior parietal bone.[50] The dissection to the parietal bone is safe and direct, passing through the layers of the SCALP (skin, subcutaneous fat, aponeurosis, loose connective tissue, and pericranium). The skull itself is composed of the outer cortex, the medullary space or diploe, and the inner cortex (**Fig. 6**).

Although the calvarial bone graft harvest is not without risk, the incidence of major complications is very small **Box 4**. Alopecia is the most common complication and can be minimized by limited cautery along the incision line. Larson[51] reported donor site morbidity in a series of 89 patients undergoing graft harvest. All of their grafts were procured from the parietal-occipital region through either a coronal incision or through a linear incision directly over the harvest site. They encountered two patients with inadequate bone thickness to harvest a split thickness graft, which resulted in dural exposure without dural tear or bleeding. One patient developed a postoperative hematoma. Preoperative radiographic evaluation can help avoid a dural tear. Posterior-anterior and lateral skull films are suggested as a minimal preoperative study. However, cone beam or CT scans can more accurately and reliably measure cranial bone thickness.[52] In a series of 33 patients undergoing calvarial bone graft, Harsha and colleagues[53] reported three instances of perforation of the inner cortex,

one of which required primary closure of a dural tear. Cannella and Hopkins[54] reported a laceration of the superior sagittal sinus while harvesting an outer table graft. Other potential complications include injury to the middle meningeal artery resulting in an epidural hematoma.

There are multiple ways to exploit the ample amount of bone available in the calvarium. Harvest techniques can be divided into split outer-table grafts (partial thickness of outer cortex), outer-table grafts (full thickness of outer cortex), split bicortical grafts, and full-thickness bicortical grafts. Stevens and Heit[55] described a technique of harvesting large, full-thickness outer-table cranial bone grafts using the Gigli saw. After standard exposure, they outlined the graft with a fissure bur into the diploe. They then elevated the outer perimeter of the graft site with a large acrylic bur, followed by outer-table removal with the Gigli saw. They described this technique as advantageous over other split-thickness techniques as it facilitates the harvest of large pieces of outer-table bone, it shortens the operation time, it decreases the chance of graft fracture, and it virtually eliminates inner-table perforation or fracture caused by osteotomes. The reported disadvantages of this technique were that it requires a larger soft tissue reflection and that there is a learning curve for those with limited experience using a Gigli saw. Multiple minimally invasive techniques have also been described. An in-office harvest was described by using a bone scraper to collect bone shavings in which up to 14 cc of bone was harvested.[56] Similarly, particulate bone can be collected using an oval bur and a suction equipped with a bone trap.[49]

COMPARATIVE MORBIDITY

In the most extensive comparative donor site morbidity review to date, Tessier and colleagues[57] reported their combined complication rate of each of the major bone graft donor sites in their group experience of 20,000 cases. Iliac crest complications included six hematomas, one hernia, 10 paresthesias, eight broken figure-of-8 wires requiring removal, and two retained sponges requiring removal. In total, they experienced 27 complications of 5600 cases (0.5 percent). Tibial bone graft complications included one fracture, one late bleed, and one infection; thus three complications of 950 cases (0.3 percent). Cranial bone grafts resulted in 12 hematomas or seromas, one retained sponge, two infections, nine dural lacerations requiring suture, and three neurologic sequelae, all transient (one hemiparesis, one leg weakness, and the other

Box 4
Complications associated with calvarial graft harvest
Alopecia
Hematoma
Dural tear
Superior sagital sinus laceration
Epidural hematoma
Infection
Scarring

unspecified). These totaled 27 complications in 10,550 cases (0.3%).

FUTURE INVESTIGATIONS

Boyne and Herford[58] suggested an algorithm for alveolar reconstruction before implant placement based on the size and geometry of the defect. Regardless of the source of bone graft, the long-term stability of the graft under function is paramount to a successful treatment. As in-office cone beam technology becomes more prevalent, clinical researchers will be able to better quantify and compare the long-term success of various bone graft sources and techniques for reconstruction. One study has shown preprosthetic calvarial bone inlay and onlay grafts to have a postgrafting volume reduction of 16.2% and 19.2% at 6 months and 1 year, respectively, without a decrease in bone density.[59]

SUMMARY

With adequate training and experience, bone graft harvest from distant sites has a very low incidence of complications. A thorough understanding of the relevant anatomy, various harvest techniques, and potential morbidity associated with each harvest site will aid the surgeon in selecting the optimal bone graft source.

REFERENCES

1. Bell WH. Current concepts of bone grafting. J Oral Surg 1948;26:119–24.
2. Block MS. Horizontal ridge augmentation using particulate bone. Atlas Oral Maxillofac Surg Clin North Am 2006;14:27–38.
3. Ozaki W, Buchman SR. Volume maintenance of onlay bone grafts in the craniofacial skeleton: micro-architecture versus embryologic origin. Plast Reconstr Surg 1998;102(2):291–9.
4. Rosenthal AH, Buchman SR. Volume maintenance of inlay bone grafts in the craniofacial skeleton. Plast Reconstr Surg 2003;112(3):802–11.
5. Gbara A, Darwich K, Li Lei, et al. Long-term results of jaw reconstruction with microsurgical fibula grafts and dental implants. J Oral Maxillofac Surg 2007;65:1005–9.
6. Ebraheim NA, Yang H, Lu J, et al. Anterior iliac crest bone graft. Anatomic considerations. Spine 1997;22(8):847–9.
7. Beirne JC, Barry HJ, Brady FA, et al. Donor site morbidity of the anterior iliac crest following cancellous bone harvest. Int J Oral Maxillofac Surg 1996;25:268–71.
8. Kademani D, Keller E. Iliac crest grafting for mandibular reconstruction. Atlas Oral Maxillofac Surg Clin North Am 2006;14:161–70.
9. Chou D, Storm PB, Campbell JN. Vulnerability of the subcostal nerve to injury during bone graft harvesting from the iliac crest. J Neurosurg 2004;1:87–9.
10. Aszmann OC, Dellon ES, Dellon AL. Anatomical course of the lateral femoral cutaneous nerve and its susceptibility to compression and injury. Plast Reconstr Surg 1997;100(3):600–4.
11. Mischkowski RA, Selbach I, Neugebauer J, et al. Lateral femoral cutaneous nerve and iliac crest bone grafts—anatomical and clinical considerations. Int J Oral Maxillofac Surg 2006;35:366–72.
12. Tayapongsak P, Wimsatt JA, LaBanc JP, et al. Morbidity from anterior ilium bone harvest. A comparative study of lateral versus medial surgical approach. Oral Surg Oral Med Oral Pathol 1994;78(3):296–300.
13. Falkensammer N, Kirmeier R, Arnetzl C, et al. Modified iliac bone harvesting—morbidity and patients' experience. J Oral Maxillofac Surg 2009;67:1700–5.
14. Grillon GL, Gunther SF, Connole PW. A new technique for obtaining iliac bone grafts. J Oral Maxillofac Surg 1984;42(3):172–6.
15. Bapat MR, Chaudhary K, Garg H, et al. Reconstruction of large iliac crest defects after graft harvest using autogenous rib graft: a prospective controlled study. Spine 2008;33(23):2570–5.
16. Resnick DK. Reconstruction of anterior iliac crest after bone graft harvest decreases pain: a randomized, controlled clinical trial. Neurosurgery 2005;57(3):526–9.
17. De Riu G, Meloni SM, Raho MT, et al. Delayed iliac abscess as an unusual complication of an iliac bone graft in an orthognathic case. Int J Oral Maxillofac Surg 2008;37:1156–8.
18. Zijderveld SA, Bruggenkate CM, van Den Bergh JP, et al. Fractures of the iliac crest after split-thickness bone grafting for preprosthetic surgery: report of 3 cases and review of the literature. J Oral Maxillofac Surg 2004;62:781–6.
19. Bloomquist DS, Feldman GR. The posterior ilium as a donor site for maxilla-facial bone grafting. J Maxillofac Surg 1980;8(1):60–4.
20. Xu R, Ebraheim NA, Yeasting RA, et al. Anatomic considerations for posterior iliac bone harvesting. Spine 1996;21(9):1017–20.
21. Marx RE. Bone harvest from the posterior ilium. Atlas Oral Maxillofac Surg Clin North Am 2005;13:109–18.
22. Kim DH, Rhim R, Li L, et al. Prospective study of iliac crest bone graft harvest site pain and morbidity. Spine J 2009;9(11):886–92.
23. Schwartz CE, Martha JF, Kowalski P, et al. Prospective evaluation of chronic pain associated with

posterior autologous iliac crest bone graft harvest and its effect on postoperative outcome. Health Qual Life Outcomes 2009;7:49.

24. Hall MB, Vallerand WP, Thompson D, et al. Comparative anatomic study of anterior and posterior iliac crests as donor sites. J Oral Maxillofac Surg 1991; 49:560–3.

25. Marx RE, Morales MJ. Morbidity from bone harvest in major jaw reconstruction: a randomized trial comparing the lateral anterior and posterior approaches to the ilium. J Oral Maxillofac Surg 1988;48:196–203.

26. Kessler P, Thorwarth M, Bloch-Birkholz A, et al. Harvesting of bone from the iliac crest: comparison of the anterior and posterior sites. Br J Oral Maxillofac Surg 2005;43:51–6.

27. Nkenke E, Weisbach V, Winckler E, et al. Morbidity of harvesting of bone grafts from the iliac crest for preprosthetic augmentation procedures: a prospective study. Int J Oral Maxillofac Surg 2004;33:157–63.

28. Nocini PF, Bedogni A, Valsecchi S, et al. Fractures of the iliac crest following anterior and posterior bone graft harvesting. Review of the literature and case presentation. Minerva Stomatol 2003; 52(10):441–52.

29. O'Keeffe RM, Riemer BL, Butterfield SL. Harvesting of autogenous cancellous bone graft from the proximal tibial metaphysis. A review of 230 cases. J Orthop Trauma 1991;5(4):469–74.

30. Catone GA, Reimer BL, McNeir D, et al. Tibia-autogenous cancellous bone as an alternative donor site in maxillofacial surgery: a preliminary report. J Oral Maxillofac Surg 1992;50:1256–63.

31. Wang K, Almeida LE, Olsson AB. Volume analysis of the proximal tibial metaphysis. J Oral Maxillofac Surg 2007;65:2425–9.

32. Sivarajasingam V, Pell G, Morse M, et al. Secondary bone grafting of alveolar clefts: a densitometric comparison of iliac crest and tibial bone grafts. Cleft Palate Craniofac J 2001;38:11–4.

33. Kushner GM. Tibia bone graft harvest technique. Atlas Oral Maxillofac Surg Clin North Am 2005;13: 119–26.

34. Herford AS, King BJ, Audia F, et al. Medial approach for tibial bone graft: anatomic study and clinical technique. J Oral Maxillofac Surg 2003;61:358–63.

35. Jakse N, Seibert FJ, Lorenzoni M, et al. A modified technique of harvesting tibial cancellous bone and its use for sinus grafting. Clin Oral Implants Res 2001;12:488–94.

36. Lezcano FJ, Cagigal BP, Cantera JM, et al. Technical note: medial approach for proximal tibia bone graft using a manual trephine. Oral Surg Oral Med Oral Pathol Oral Radiol Endod 2007; 104:11–7.

37. van Damme PA, Merkx MA. A modification of the tibial bone graft harvesting technique. Int J Oral Maxillofac Surg 1996;25:346–8.

38. Hashemi HM. Oblique use of a trephine bur for the harvesting of tibial bone grafts. Br J Oral Maxillofac Surg 2008;46:690–1.

39. Alfaro FH, Marti C, Biosca MJ, et al. Minimally invasive tibial bone harvesting under intravenous sedation. J Oral Maxillofac Surg 2005;63:464–70.

40. Marchena JM, Block MS, Stover JD. Tibial bone harvesting under intravenous sedation: morbidity and patient experiences. J Oral Maxillofac Surg 2002; 60:1151–4.

41. Kirmeir R, Payer M, Lorenzoni M, et al. Harvesting of cancellous bone from the proximal tibia under local anesthesia: donor site morbidity and patient experience. J Oral Maxillofac Surg 2007; 65:2235–41.

42. Schmidt ER, Townsend J. Unusual complication of subacute osteomyelitis following tibial bone graft: report of a case. J Oral Maxillofac Surg 2008;66: 1290–3.

43. Alt V, Nawab A, Seligson D. Bone grafting from the proximal tibia. J Trauma 1999;47(3):555–7.

44. Hughes CW, Peter J, Revington PJ. The proximal tibia donor site in cleft alveolar bone grafting: experience of 75 consecutive cases. J Craniomaxillofac Surg 2002;30(1):12–6.

45. Thor A, Farzad P, Larsson S. Fracture of the tibia: complication of bone grafting to the anterior maxilla. Br J Oral Maxillofac Surg 2006;44:46–8.

46. Bottlang M. Effect of tibial graft harvest on plateau compliance: a biomechanical study. J Oral Maxillofac Surg 2008;66(8):52.

47. Ilankovan V, Stronczek M, Telfer M, et al. A prospective study of trephined bone grafts of the tibial shaft and iliac crest. Br J Oral Maxillofac Surg 1998;36:434–9.

48. Tessier P. Autogenous bone grafts taken from the calvarium for facial and cranial applications. Clin Plast Surg 1982;9:531–8.

49. Ruiz RL, Turvey TA, Costello BJ, et al. Cranial bone grafts: craniomaxillofacial applications and harvesting techniques. Atlas Oral Maxillofac Surg Clin North Am 2005;13:127–37.

50. Gonzalez AM, Papay FE, Zins JE. Calvarial thickness and its relation to cranial bone harvest. Plast Reconstr Surg 2006;117(6):1964–71.

51. Larson PE. Morbidity associated with calvarial bone graft harvest. J Oral Maxillofac Surg 1989; 47(8):110–1.

52. Tellioglu AT, Yilmaz S, Baydar S, et al. Computed tomographic evaluation before cranial bone harvesting to avoid unexpected hazards during aesthetic procedures. Aesthetic Plast Surg 2001;25:198–201.

53. Harsha BC, Turvey TA, Powers SK. Use of autogenous cranial bone grafts in maxillofacial surgery:

a preliminary report. J Oral Maxillofac Surg 1966;44: 11–5.

54. Cannella DM, Hopkins LN. Superior sagittal sinus laceration complicating an autogenous calvarial bone graft harvest: report of a case. J Oral Maxillofac Surg 1990;48:741–3.

55. Stevens MR, Heit JM. Calvarial bone graft harvest using the Gigli saw. J Oral Maxillofac Surg 1998; 56:798–9.

56. Al-Sebaei MO, Papageorge MB, Woo T. Technique for in-office cranial bone harvesting. J Oral Maxillofac Surg 2004;62:120–2.

57. Tessier P, Kawamoto H, Posnick J, et al. Complications of harvesting autogenous bone grafts: a group experience of 20,000 cases. Plast Reconstr Surg 2005;166:72–3.

58. Boyne PJ, Herford AS. An algorithm for reconstruction of alveolar defects before implant placement. Oral Maxillofac Surg Clin North Am 2001;13(3): 533–41.

59. Smolka W, Eggensperger N, Carollo V, et al. Changes in the volume and density of calvarial split bone grafts after alveolar ridge augmentation. Clin Oral Implants Res 2006;17(2):149–55.

Bone Graft Harvesting from Regional Sites

Somsak Sittitavornwong, DDS, MS, DMD[a],*,
Rajesh Gutta, BDS, MS[b]

KEYWORDS

- Mandibular symphysis • Osteotomy • Grafting • Implant

Successful osseointegration of dental implants requires sufficient bone surrounding the implant. Although bone substitutes and augmentation techniques offer viable prognoses for achieving the required amount of hard tissue augmentation, autologous bone is the gold standard with regard to quantity, quality, and an uneventful healing.

The limitation of using autologous bone is harvesting adequate bone for reconstruction without exceeding acceptable donor site morbidity. The choice of donor site depends largely on the quality, quantity, and form of the bone required. The amount of time required and the accessibility of the donor site must also be considered. Intraoral bone harvesting has the advantage of being performed in the same operative field and being carried out on an outpatient basis with the patient under local anesthesia.

Intramembranous bone is thought to undergo less resorption than endochondral bone. The calvaria, maxillary bones, and mandibular body and ramus are of intramembranous origin, whereas the mandibular condyles are of endochondral origin.[1] The mandibular donor site is one of the alternative sources of membranous bone, which is thought to undergo less resorption than endochondral bone.[2–10] In addition to quick bone harvesting with minimal morbidity, the intraoral bone harvesting techniques do not cause cutaneous scarring. The advantages of using mandibular donor site for bone grafting are increased bone volume and quality (bone density) of recipient site. Increased bone density of the

recipient site is replicated from symphysis (bone density D-1 and D-2) or ramus (D-I) as donor sites with minimal bone resorption (0%–20%).[11] Different autologous-bone donor sites can serve this purpose. Small bone blocks harvested from the mandibular body, ascending ramus, symphysis, or posterior maxillary region are common donor sites. Vital anatomy such as teeth, maxillary sinuses, and mental and inferior alveolar nerves must be considered and can limit intraoral bone harvesting techniques. Alternative sources for local harvesting in the mandible can be evaluated by careful clinical and radiographic examinations of the patient. Tori and alveolar exostoses are common, suitable, alternative intraoral bone sources.

CLINICAL AND SCIENTIFIC BACKGROUND OF INTRAORAL AUTOGENOUS BONE HARVESTING
Mandibular Symphysis

Alveolar bone grafts for dental implants are indicated when the height of the alveolar crest is usually less than 5 mm or the width is less than 4 mm. The quantity and quality of donor bone site should be considered when selecting the site for bone harvesting. The mandibular block grafts make the bone density of recipient bone to be advantageous over guided bone regeneration. **Table 1** shows the dimensions of bone from different locations of maxilla and mandible. The mandibular symphysis is the most available

[a] Department of Oral and Maxillofacial Surgery, University of Alabama at Birmingham, 1530 Third Avenue South, SDB 419, Birmingham, AL 35294-0007, USA
[b] Department of Oral and Maxillofacial Surgery, University of Texas Health Science Center, MSC 7908, 7703 Floyd Curl Drive, San Antonio, TX 78229, USA
* Corresponding author.
E-mail address: sjade@uab.edu

Oral Maxillofacial Surg Clin N Am 22 (2010) 317–330
doi:10.1016/j.coms.2010.04.006
1042-3699/10/$ – see front matter. Published by Elsevier Inc.

Table 1
Comparing the dimensions of intraoral bone donor sites

Donor Sites	Size of Corticocancellous Block	Volume (mL)	References
Symphysis	$20.9 \times 9.9 \times 6.9$ mm^3	4.71	Montazem et al, 2000[12]
Ascending Ramus	$37.6 \times 33.17 \times 22.48 \times 9.15$ mm^4	2.36	Gungormus and Yavuz, 2002[13]
Lateral Ramus	1.3 cm $\times 3$ cm^2	NA	Li and Schwartz, 1996[14]
Coronoid Process	$18 \times 17 \times 5$ mm^3	NA	Choung and Kim, 2001[15]
Zygomatic Buttress	1.5×2.0 cm^2	NA	Gellrich et al, 2007[16]

Abbreviation: NA, not applicable.

source of bone graft. The amount of bone available for harvesting is sufficient for defects measuring up to the width of 3 teeth. Predictability of bone augmentation from the symphysis is up to 6 mm in horizontal and vertical dimensions.

There are 2 incision designs for mandibular symphysis harvest (**Fig. 1**). One is sulcular incision and another is vestibular incision. Care must be exercised with regard to proximity of the mental nerves. The sulcular incision is considered in cases with healthy periodontium or no anterior crowns, which could initiate gingival recession. The oblique releasing incision can be made at a distal line angle of the second lower premolar. The vestibular incision causes more bleeding from the mentalis muscle but provides less access than the sulcular incision.

The vestibular incision is similar to a genioplasty approach (**Fig. 2**) in which the incision is made through the mentalis muscle and preserves the gingival, periosteal, and mentalis insertion attachments superior to the chin. The incision is closed in 2 layers, thus preventing mentalis or chin ptosis. The vestibular incision is associated with wound dehiscence (11%), scar band formation, more pain, and possible chin ptosis compared with sulcular incision.[11]

For harvesting a mandibular symphysis graft, the superior osteotomy line should be made at least 5 mm below the root apices (**Fig. 3**). An osteotomy in the mandibular symphyseal region should completely penetrate the labial cortical plate. Its final depth depends on the thickness of the graft required. A free bone block graft is generally harvested in the form of a corticocancellous bone block.

Mandibular Ramus and Body

Li and Schwartz[14] determined that the average bone size obtained from the lateral plate of the mandibular body was 1.5×3 cm (**Fig. 4**). The thickness of mandibular ramus provides only cortical bone, which ranges from 2 to 4.5 mm. Most sites

provide a thickness of 3 to 4 mm. The mandibular ramus has adequate bone volume measuring up to 3-tooth and even 4-tooth edentulous site for grafting. The bone density of mandibular ramus is D-1. Predictability of bone augmentation is up to 3 to 4 mm in horizontal and vertical dimensions.

Incision for mandibular ramus bone harvesting is made distal to the most posterior tooth and continues up the ascending ramus, stripping off the temporalis muscle (**Fig. 5**). An oblique release incision into buccinator muscle may be used as needed. Three complete osteotomies are made: 1 superior and 2 vertical. Another horizontal bone groove is made at the inferior border. The superior osteotomy is made 4 to 5 mm medial to the external oblique ridge with a small fissure bur from the first or second molar region in the mandible and continues posteriorly in the ascending ramus depending on the required size. The anterior and posterior vertical osteotomies are made 10 to 12 mm in length in the superoinferior direction. Then, a groove connecting the inferior aspect of each vertical osteotomy is made. The harvest is made using a small flat chisel to complete the osteotomies. The mandibular ramus bone is carefully split from the donor site. The inferior alveolar nerve was reported to be visible in about 10% to 12% of patients.[11] The block graft is placed and secured with microscrews (**Fig. 6**). Placement of dental implants is considered 4 months after bone grafting (**Fig. 7**).

Complications of bone harvesting from mandibular symphysis and ramus are variable. Clavero and Lundgren[17] reported that temporary mental nerve hypesthesia was about 76% in the symphysis group and 21% in the ascending ramus group. After 18 months, 52% of the symphysis group still had decreased sensitivity and permanent altered sensation, whereas the ascending ramus group had only 3% of decreased sensitivity with permanent altered sensation in the posterior vestibular area. Pikos[18] stated that infection rates after bone harvesting from mandibular symphysis

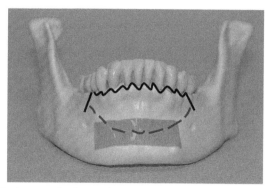

Fig. 1. Harvesting of mandibular symphysis can be approached by vestibular (*red line*) or sulcular incisions (*black line*).

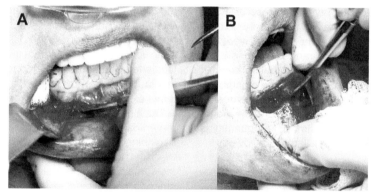

Fig. 2. Vestibular incision was made approximately 1.5 cm from the gingival sulcus (*A*). Labial bone cortex of mandibular symphysis is displayed (*B*).

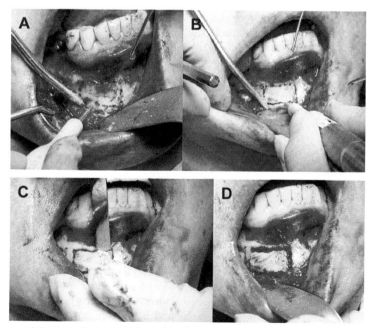

Fig. 3. The osteotomy of the mandibular symphyseal region was marked by penetrating a small round and fissure bur at the labial cortical plate (*A, B*). A thin chisel was used for completing the osteotomy (*C*). A free bone block graft was harvested in the form of a corticocancellous bone block (*D*).

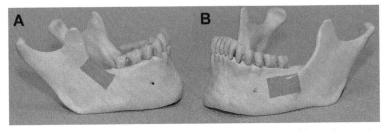

Fig. 4. Ascending mandibular ramus (*A*) and body (*B*) can be other sources of bone harvesting.

and ramus are minimal (<1%). Permanent neurosensory deficits after bone harvesting from mandibular symphysis and ramus is less than 1%. Postoperative trismus after ramus bone harvesting is high (approximately 60%) but transient and can take up to 3 to 4 weeks to resolve. Postoperative morbidity, mainly temporary paresthesia, differs among the sites used for harvesting: for the chin it ranges from 10% to 50%,[17,19] whereas for the mandibular ramus it ranges from 0% to 5%.[17,19] Thus, the mandibular ramus has some advantages when compared with the mental symphysis as a possible donor site: the quality of bone is similar, the quantity is more, and the risk of neural damage is lower.[20]

Mandibular Coronoid Process

Mandibular coronoid bone grafting was introduced in 1969 for the repair of small discontinuity defects of the mandible (**Fig. 8**).[21] The technique is fairly quick and simple. It can be done on an outpatient basis. The coronoid process is a membranous bone with a thick cortical region. The bone density of coronoid process is D-1.

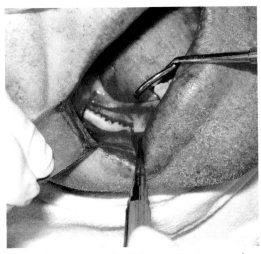

Fig. 5. The osteotomy for right mandibular ramus harvesting was performed for reconstruction of vertical mandibular body atrophy.

Choung and Kim[15] reported that the thickness of the coronoid process was similar to that of the calvarial bone, which ranges from 4 to 7 mm. The lingula is usually located 10 mm or more below the sigmoid notch. Therefore, the region 5 mm below the sigmoid notch may be safely used without damage to the inferior alveolar neurovascular bundles. The coronoid process has adequate bone volume for up to 1-tooth and 2-tooth edentulous sites. Predictability of bone augmentation is up to 3 to 4 mm in horizontal and vertical dimensions.

The left lateral coronoid process is accessed via a vertical incision over the ascending ramus, beginning at the level of the occlusal surface of the last molar and extending to the midpoint of the ramus. The temporalis muscle is completely stripped and dissected from its attachment. The coronoid process is stabilized with bone forceps during cutting with a reciprocating saw or drill. The coronoid process graft is set aside in normal saline, and the incision is closed.

The coronoid process bone graft offers several advantages including no facial scarring, no devitalization of the dentition, ease of access, and superior bone quality. Choung and Kim[15] did not observe any complication or permanent mortality in the donor site after harvesting coronoid process. No significant functional limitations were reported.

ZYGOMATIC BUTTRESS

The zygomatic buttress is a donor site that offers easy access with excellent visibility and yields good quality bone of correct morphology (**Fig. 9**). The zygomatic buttress is a strong bony support that provides pressure absorption in the midfacial skeleton. A bone graft of 1.5 to 2 cm^2 taken from the caudal zygomatic buttress zone can be harvested with minimal donor site morbidity.[16] However, the bone quantity from this site is limited and is suitable only for small bony defects. This donor site might be adequate to reconstruct alveolar defects of 1- and 2-tooth edentulous site. The bone density of zygomatic buttress is D-1 to D-2.

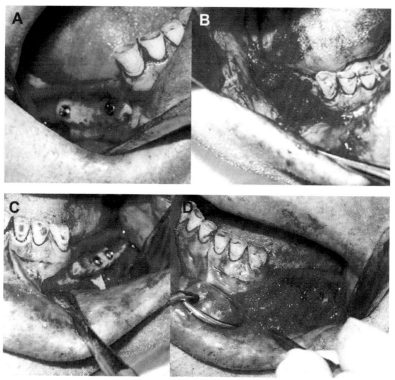

Fig. 6. Right and left ramus bone grafts were placed and secured with 2 microscrews on each side of the mandibular body to increase vertical and horizontal atrophy (*A, C*). Additional particulate graft was used over the ramus block graft (*B, D*).

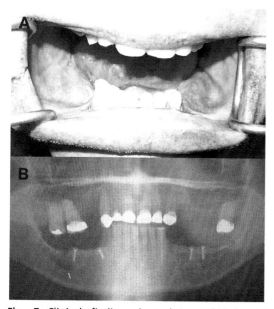

Fig. 7. Clinical finding showed normal intraoral wound healing (*A*). Panoramic radiograph showed a good position of block graft and microscrews 4 months after surgery (*B*).

Predictability of bone augmentation is up to 3 to 4 mm in horizontal and vertical dimensions.

The zygomatic buttress is accessed by vestibular incision along the buccal aspect from canine to first molar teeth (**Fig. 10**). The mucobuccal flap is reflected in a superolateral direction. The infraorbital nerve is identified and secured. The anterior and lateral aspects of zygomatic buttress are visualized. Four complete osteotomies are made with a small fissure bur: 2 horizontal and 2 vertical. The superior and inferior vertical osteotomies of 10 to 12 mm in length are made in the superoinferior direction at the donor site. The complete osteotomy is made by using a small flat chisel. The zygomatic buttress graft is carefully split from the donor site. The schneiderian membrane is usually visible. Maxillary sinus elevators can be used for detaching maxillary mucosa from the bone graft. The bone graft is preserved in normal saline, and the incision is closed in the usual manner. Placement of a dental implant can be considered 4 months after bone grafting (**Fig. 11**).

After bone harvesting from this area, postoperative trismus as well as injury to the adjacent soft tissues with hemorrhage can occur. Limiting factors are the mucous membrane of the adjacent

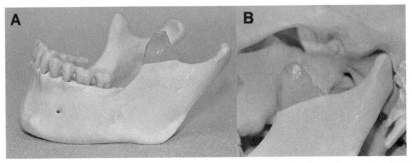

Fig. 8. Mandibular coronoid process has approximately 15 × 15 × 5 mm for bone harvesting (*A, B*).

maxillary sinus and the close relationship to the infraorbital foramen. However, direct visualization of the infraorbital region allows nerve identification and preservation during bone graft harvesting. The mucous membrane of the adjacent maxillary sinus can be visualized and involved in graft harvesting site. Ideally, the patient should not have any sinus problems. As an additional caution, use of ultrasound-based dissection with piezosurgery might further reduce the danger of perforating the sinus membrane.[22–24]

ALVEOLAR RECONSTRUCTION WITH INTRAORAL BONE GRAFTS

Severe alveolar bone resorption or pneumatization of the maxillary sinus makes it difficult to perform the conventional dental implantation procedure. Several techniques of alveolar reconstruction have been innovated, including interpositioning bone graft (sandwich osteotomies), vertical or horizontal onlay bone graft, and particulate bone graft with and without guided tissue regeneration

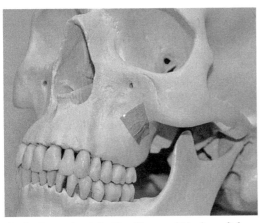

Fig. 9. Approximately 15 × 20 mm of block graft from zygomatic buttress can be harvested.

membrane. Most techniques try to correct alveolar bone defects before implant placement.

INTERPOSITIONING BONE GRAFT (SANDWICH OSTEOTOMIES)

In 1970s, Schettler and Holtermann[25] first proposed a sandwich technique for mandibular alveolar ridge augmentation. In 1980s, Obwegeser and Farmand[26] first reported a horseshoe-sandwich osteotomy of the severe atrophic edentulous maxilla. Farmand[27] used the horseshoe sandwich osteotomy of the edentulous maxilla with interposition of iliac crest or ribs in combination with a modified submucous vestibuloplasty for preprosthetic surgery. The vertical resorption rate was found to be 1.8 mm (20%) after 3 years, with 93% of cases (28 out of 30) revealing satisfactory results in clinical investigation.[27] The technique of interpositional bone graft has been modified for increasing vertical dimension of the severe atrophic maxilla and mandible.

The advantages of sandwich osteotomies in the maxilla include interdental papillary support, no significant bone resorption before implant placement and more stable augmentation than onlay bone grafting, and gain in vertical dimension in the esthetic zone.[8] Sandwich osteotomies can be performed anywhere in the arches but is perhaps most indicated in the esthetic zone such as anterior maxilla. The alveolar segment can be mobilized and fixated to increase vertical dimension of up to 8 mm in the posterior mandible and 5 mm in the anterior maxilla.[28,29]

The incision design for the recipient site varies with the location within the arches. The vestibular incision is designed for approaching the recipient site and remains up to 10 mm away from the crest (**Figs. 12** and **13**). This preserves the blood supply to osteotomized alveolar segment. Buccal flap is reflected enough to make 2 vertical and 1 horizontal osteotomies with a fine fissure bur or sagittal saw. A horizontal cut is made

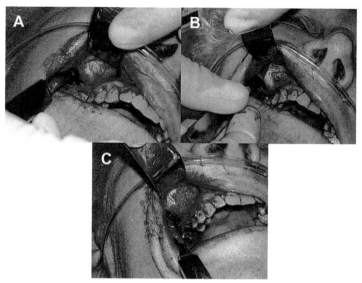

Fig. 10. Hemi-Le Fort I incision was made for the access (*A*). The bone graft was harvested from right zygomatic buttress, and right maxillary sinus lift was performed simultaneously for reconstruction of edentulous area number 3 (*B*). Additional particulate graft was placed in the recipient site (*C*).

approximately 5 mm below the crest of the alveolar ridge. Two slightly divergent vertical osteotomies are connected by the horizontal cut and alveolar crest to free the alveolar segment. The alveolar segment may be 3-tooth to 6-tooth edentulous site in length, inclusive of the incisor region. If the posterior mandible is the operation site, the mental nerve is identified and secured. The horizontal osteotomy is approached to within 2 mm of the inferior alveolar nerve. The osteotomy is proceeded lateromedially until through the lingual plate. An osteotome can be used to free the segment.

A miniplate might be used to stabilize the segment vertically. The alveolar crest can be widened with an oblique alveolar osteotomy (**Fig. 14**). This widening could change the narrow edge of the alveolar bone to a wider ridge. The block graft is wedged and placed between the segment and the basal bone followed by the addition of particulate autograft. In most instances, the cortical wedge of bone is adequate for stability of the alveolar segment without miniplate and screws. After that the wound is closed in the regular fashion. After 4 months of healing, dental implant placement using a guide stent can be proceeded in a standard

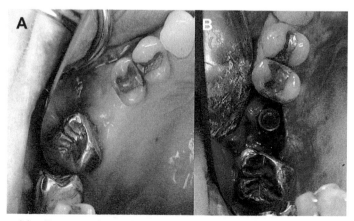

Fig. 11. Normal wound healing was observed (*A*). A dental implant was placed at the reconstruction site 4 months after bone grafting (*B*).

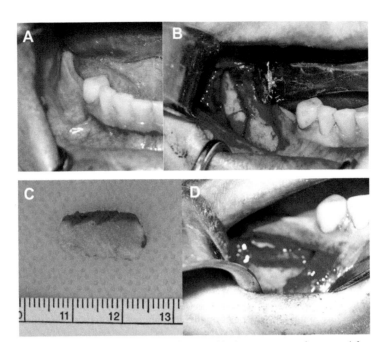

Fig. 12. Atrophic right mandibular body (*A*). The right mandibular ramus was harvested for sandwich graft (*B*). Block bone graft from right mandibular ramus was measured (*C*). The block graft was placed in the osteotomy site for gaining the vertical dimension (*D*).

fashion. Implant placement shortly after graft incorporation has a stimulating effect on the bone, preserving the augmented bone volume and preventing further loss.

VERTICAL OR HORIZONTAL ONLAY BONE GRAFT

After tooth loss, the alveolar process undergoes a progressive, irreversible resorption, resulting in

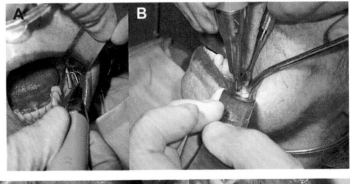

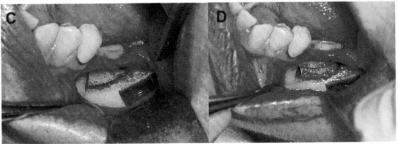

Fig. 13. Peizosurgery can be used for intraoral bone harvesting with good hemostasis and low risk of nerve injury during osteotomy (*A, B*). The left mandibular ramus is harvested and placed in the osteotomy site at the left mandibular body (*C, D*).

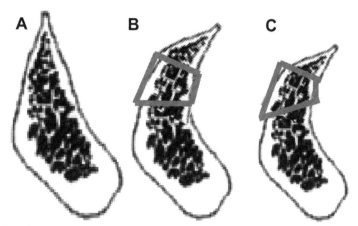

Fig. 14. Knife alveolar edge is usually observed a long time after tooth loss (*A*). The horizontal osteotomy is made and sandwich graft is placed (*B*). The angle osteotomy can be made for gaining the width of the alveolar crest after placement of sandwich graft (*C*).

loss of bony substance both vertically and horizontally. The use of bone from the mandibular symphysis, retromolar area, mandibular ramus, and the maxillary tuberosity can serve as a good treatment alternative for alveolar ridge augmentation. Additional bone improves the supporting quality of dental implants by decreasing the crown-to-implant ratio. Good-quality bone after augmentation allows the clinician to place a wider and longer implant. The alveolar ridge should have adequate width to allow bone on both facial and lingual implant surfaces for circumferential osseointegration. Cortical bone grafts maintain their volumes significantly better than cancellous bone grafts.[30] Less resorption of this bone makes it more favorable for implant placement.

Incision design at the recipient site for block grafting varies depending on the location within the arches. The cortical bone graft can be placed on the lateral or vertical aspect of the alveolar ridge. The recipient site should be prepared to allow the block graft to fit as an inlay graft. The block graft is usually stabilized with 1 to 2 titanium microscrews of 1.5 mm in diameter (**Fig. 15**). In case the recipient site is a long span, 2 fixation screws protect the rotation of the block graft. The length of the recipient site does not influence the outcome.[31] Demineralized bone can be added around and between the block graft and recipient site. The intraoral block bone graft procedure can be combined with other surgical procedures, such as sinus lift elevation or nasal floor elevation. Successful treatment of localized ridge defects can be achieved with autologous intraoral bone transplant with and without combined–guided bone regeneration. Jensen and colleagues[32] found that combined use of bone grafts and

membranes had less resorption of autologous block grafts when membranes were used in a canine model. In addition, graft surface resorption of autologous onlay block bone grafts is reduced in alveolar crest augmentation when the grafts are protected by regeneration membranes.[33,34] In contrast, autografts without membrane protection showed considerable crestal bone resorption.[34] After graft incorporation, implants can be placed either submerged or nonsubmerged, depending on relative density of the overall recipient site.

SOCKET GRAFTING

The healing of extraction socket involves a series of physiologic events including formation of coagulum that was replaced with (1) a connective tissue matrix in 1 month, (2) an immature bone that fills up the socket in 3 months, and (3) a cortical ridge that includes woven and lamellar bone. This socket is gradually replaced by lamellar bone and marrow.[35] Placement of implants into fresh extraction sockets is not always possible. Improper implant placement can lead to esthetic disasters, displaced interarch relationships, periodontal problems, and a potential loss of implant. Bone loss occurs in vertical and horizontal planes, with the horizontal loss exceeding vertical bone loss. As much as 60% of the alveolar width and 40% of the height may be lost in the first 6 months after tooth extraction.[36] Socket grafting has been shown to be superior in bone quantity and quality than extraction alone.[37]

A variety of protocols for socket preservation have been reported. These protocols include guided bone regeneration and bone grafts or

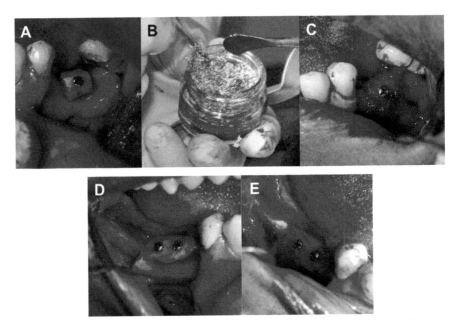

Fig. 15. An onlay graft was secured with a micropositioning screw (*A*). Particulate bone graft was mixed with autogenous blood (*B*). Additional demineralized bone was filled in the bone gaps (*C*). Vertical and horizontal onlay bone grafts were placed and fixed with microscrews (*D, E*).

a combination of both. There are 3 simple steps in socket preservation: (1) extraction of teeth, (2) placement of graft materials, and (3) tissue closure with or without membrane. After an atraumatic extraction, a graft material of choice is carefully placed into the socket without compacting tightly (**Figs. 16** and **17**). These grafts may be autografts, allografts, or xenografts. Many graft materials, including autogenous bone, demineralized freeze-dried bone allograft (DFDBA), mineralized freeze-dried bone allograft, bone allograft, bone morphogenetic protein (BMP), collagen, bovine hydroxyapatite, and alloplasts, have been evaluated in different studies for socket augmentation. Autogenous grafting is considered the gold standard. The maxillary tuberosity is an ideal site for bone harvesting for the purpose of socket grafting. This region provides adequate cancellous bone for grafting up to 2 to 3 extraction sockets. Promising results have been reported in many studies, but the search for the ideal technique and materials remains.

A randomized, masked, placebo-controlled multicenter clinical study demonstrated that the novel combination of recombinant human BMP-2 and a commonly used collagen sponge used in socket augmentation had a striking effect on de novo osseous formation for the placement of dental implants.[38] In a case series, 3 commercially available bone biomaterials were evaluated to compare their ability to allow guided bone regeneration. It was concluded that early implant osseointegration was not influenced by the application of bone biomaterials used in this study.[39] Allografts seem to perform well when compared with xenografts.[40]

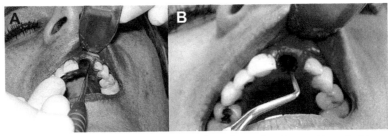

Fig. 16. A minimally traumatic technique for extraction of tooth number 9 was attempted by using a periosteotome (*A*). The socket was cleansed with a dental curette (*B*).

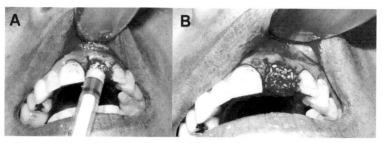

Fig. 17. The oragraft (LifeNet Health Inc, Virginia Beach, VA, USA) was placed (*A*) and condensed (*B*) into the socket of tooth number 9.

Although there are several reports indicating that socket grafting produces superior results, there have been some studies indicating that bovine bone, DFDBA, and intraoral autologous bone do not promote extraction socket healing.[41]

Bone graft, by itself, should be able to promote bone ingrowth. However, because of the nature of the extraction socket, most bone grafts may be lost if no protection is provided. Most studies advocate the superiority of combining grafts with barrier membranes than the single use of either of them. A barrier membrane may help protect the blood clot that serves as a matrix for bone formation and allows for bone regeneration. Membranes can minimize the amount of graft resorption and also eliminate the unwanted fibrous cells that compete with the osteoblasts. These membranes are helpful in stabilizing the graft material and improve the success of regeneration.[42] The choice between a resorbable and non-resorbable barrier depends mostly on the amount of time for which it is planned to stay in situ. Generally, adequate time must be given to regenerate the required bone mass. Reduced amount of autogenous bone, fewer bony walls, and larger grafts retard the period of osseoreplacement. It is suggested that the use of resorbable barriers should be limited to the cases in which their effect is required for less than 3 months. Longer healing periods entail a nonresorbable membrane. Whenever the crestal height of the socket walls are compromised, use of a titanium-reinforced membrane may be advantageous to restore the space necessary for the regeneration of the full height and width of the alveolar bone. In 1999, Sclar[43] had introduced the successful Bio-Col technique for socket preservation. The use of collagen wound dressing material was suggested not only to protect the graft materials but also to induce blood clot formation and stabilize the wound (**Figs. 18–20**). A detailed description of various barrier membranes is beyond the scope of this article.

Membranes are prone to exposure, and if it happens within the first 6 to 8 weeks of healing, the site can be rinsed out daily with 12% chlorhexidine oral rinse. Sometimes soft tissue dehiscence associated with membrane exposure may lead to pain, inflammation, swelling, and abscess. Prudent removal of the membrane and debridement of the site minimizes the risk of graft loss and further complication. In such cases, the amount of gain is invariably reduced and might need additional grafting for successful implant placement. Primary closure over the membrane is necessary to prevent oral contamination and thus failure.

DISCUSSION

Bone grafts are widely used in the reconstruction of osseous defects in the oral and maxillofacial region. Autogenous bone grafts are generally obtained

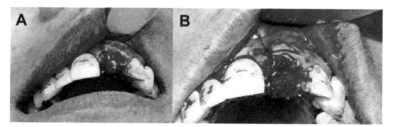

Fig. 18. CollaPlug (Zimmer Dental Inc, Carlsbad, CA, USA) was used over the allograft (*A*) and secured by resorbable suture (*B*).

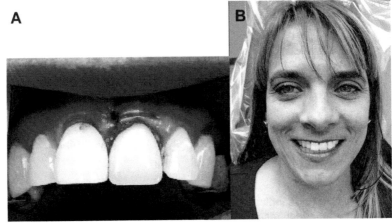

Fig. 19. A temporary upper partial denture was delivered for esthetics and gingival contouring of the soft tissue (*A, B*).

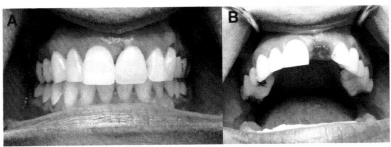

Fig. 20. Good oral hygiene was observed with a temporary upper partial denture (*A*). Normal wound healing with good gingival contour at tooth socket number 9 was observed 3 weeks after operation (*B*).

from the ilium, the rib, and the calvarium. These grafts can be easily obtained from these donor sites, but each site has associated morbidity.

The maxilla and mandible are alternative sources of membranous bone and are thought to undergo less resorption than endochondral bone. A variety of local bone grafts, such as mandibular symphysis, mandibular body, mandibular ramus, and coronoid process, have been used in oral and maxillofacial reconstruction. Intraoral bone donor sites are excellent alternatives for the augmentation of edentulous alveolar defects before implantation. Because of the quality and morphology of the bone, the alveolus can be reconstituted to its original contour. Intraoral bone can be harvested quickly with minimal morbidity. In addition, because of the intraoral approach no cutaneous scarring occurs. Thus, different sites in the mandible have been used successfully in a variety of clinical applications. However, the position of the vital anatomy including teeth, maxillary sinuses, and mental and inferior alveolar nerves must be considered and can limit intraoral

bone harvesting techniques. Alternative sources for local harvesting in the mandible can be evaluated by careful clinical and radiographic examinations of the patient.

REFERENCES

1. Nanci A, editor. Ten Cate's oral histology: development, structure, and function. 6th edition. St Louis: Mosby; 2003. p. 131–9.
2. Kusiak JF, Zins JE, Whitaker LA. The early revascularization of membranous bone. Plast Reconstr Surg 1985;76(4):510–6.
3. Hardesty RA, Marsh JL. Craniofacial onlay bone grafting: a prospective evaluation of graft morphology, orientation, and embryonic origin. Plast Reconstr Surg 1990;85(1):5–14 [discussion: 15].
4. Moskalewski S, Osiecka A, Malejczyk J. Comparison of bone formed intramuscularly after transplantation of scapular and calvarial osteoblasts. Bone 1988; 9(2):101–6.
5. Koole R, Bosker H, van der Dussen FN. Late secondary autogenous bone grafting in cleft

patients comparing mandibular (ectomesenchymal) and iliac crest (mesenchymal) grafts. J Craniomaxillofac Surg 1989;17(Suppl 1):28–30.

6. Donovan MG, Dickerson NC, Hanson LJ, et al. Maxillary and mandibular reconstruction using calvarial bone grafts and Branemark implants: a preliminary report. J Oral Maxillofac Surg 1994; 52(6):588–94.

7. Gary JJ, Donovan M, Garner FT, et al. Rehabilitation with calvarial bone grafts and osseointegrated implants after partial maxillary resection: a clinical report. J Prosthet Dent 1992;67(6):743–6.

8. Jensen J, Sindet-Pedersen S. Autogenous mandibular bone grafts and osseointegrated implants for reconstruction of the severely atrophied maxilla: a preliminary report. J Oral Maxillofac Surg 1991; 49(12):1277–87.

9. Jensen J, Sindet-Pedersen S, Oliver AJ. Varying treatment strategies for reconstruction of maxillary atrophy with implants: results in 98 patients. J Oral Maxillofac Surg 1994;52(3):210–6 [discussion: 216–8].

10. Misch CM, Misch CE. The repair of localized severe ridge defects for implant placement using mandibular bone grafts. Implant Dent 1995;4(4):261–7.

11. Alfaro FH, editor. Bone grafting in oral implantology: techniques and clinical applications. 1st edition. Barcelona, Spain: Quintessence Publishing; 2006. p. 1–234.

12. Montazem A, Valauri DV, St-Hilaire H, et al. The mandibular symphysis as a donor site in maxillofacial bone grafting: a quantitative anatomic study. J Oral Maxillofac Surg 2000;58(12):1368–71.

13. Gungormus M, Yavuz MS. The ascending ramus of the mandible as a donor site in maxillofacial bone grafting. J Oral Maxillofac Surg 2002;60(11):1316–8.

14. Li KK, Schwartz HC. Mandibular body bone in facial plastic and reconstructive surgery. Laryngoscope 1996;106(4):504–6.

15. Choung PH, Kim SG. The coronoid process for paranasal augmentation in the correction of midfacial concavity. Oral Surg Oral Med Oral Pathol Oral Radiol Endod 2001;91(1):28–33.

16. Gellrich NC, Held U, Schoen R, et al. Alveolar zygomatic buttress: a new donor site for limited preimplant augmentation procedures. J Oral Maxillofac Surg 2007;65(2):275–80.

17. Clavero J, Lundgren S. Ramus or chin grafts for maxillary sinus inlay and local onlay augmentation: comparison of donor site morbidity and complications. Clin Implant Dent Relat Res 2003; 5(3):154–60.

18. Pikos M. Mandibular block autografts for alveolar ridge augmentation. Atlas Oral Maxillofacial Surg Clin N Am 2005;13:91–107.

19. Chiapasco M, Abati S, Romeo E, et al. Clinical outcome of autogenous bone blocks or guided bone regeneration with e-PTFE membranes for the reconstruction of narrow edentulous ridges. Clin Oral Implants Res 1999;10(4):278–88.

20. Chiapasco M, Zaniboni M, Boisco M. Augmentation procedures for the rehabilitation of deficient edentulous ridges with oral implants. Clin Oral Implants Res 2006;17(Suppl 2):136–59.

21. Youmans RD, Russell EA Jr. The coronoid process: a new donor source for autogenous bone grafts. Oral Surg Oral Med Oral Pathol 1969;27(3):422–8.

22. Barone A, Santini S, Marconcini S, et al. Osteotomy and membrane elevation during the maxillary sinus augmentation procedure. A comparative study: piezoelectric device vs. conventional rotative instruments. Clin Oral Implants Res 2008;19(5):511–5.

23. Su YC. [Development and clinical application of ultrasonic osteotomy in dentistry]. Shanghai Kou Qiang Yi Xue 2007;16(1):1–7 [in Chinese].

24. Vercellotti T, De Paoli S, Nevins M. The piezoelectric bony window osteotomy and sinus membrane elevation: introduction of a new technique for simplification of the sinus augmentation procedure. Int J Periodontics Restorative Dent 2001;21(6): 561–7.

25. Schettler D, Holtermann W. Clinical and experimental results of a sandwich-technique for mandibular alveolar ridge augmentation. J Maxillofac Surg 1977;5(3):199–202.

26. Obwegeser HL, Farmand M. [Horseshoe sandwich osteotomy of the edentulous maxilla with simultaneous submucosal vestibuloplasty. A method for the advancement and deepening of the edentulous maxillary alveolar process with simultaneous elevation of the palatal arch]. Schweiz Monatsschr Zahnmed 1984;94(5):390–8 [in German].

27. Farmand M. Long-term results after horseshoe sandwich osteotomy of the edentulous maxilla as a preprosthetic procedure. J Craniomaxillofac Surg 1992;20(4):171–7.

28. Jensen OT. Alveolar segmental "sandwich" osteotomies for posterior edentulous mandibular sites for dental implants. J Oral Maxillofac Surg 2006;64(3): 471–5.

29. Jensen OT, Kuhlke L, Bedard JF, et al. Alveolar segmental sandwich osteotomy for anterior maxillary vertical augmentation prior to implant placement. J Oral Maxillofac Surg 2006;64(2):290–6.

30. Ozaki W, Buchman SR. Volume maintenance of onlay bone grafts in the craniofacial skeleton: micro-architecture versus embryologic origin. Plast Reconstr Surg 1998;102(2):291–9.

31. Schwartz-Arad D, Levin L. Intraoral autogenous block onlay bone grafting for extensive reconstruction of atrophic maxillary alveolar ridges. J Periodontol 2005;76(4):636–41.

32. Jensen OT, Greer RO Jr, Johnson L, et al. Vertical guided bone-graft augmentation in a new canine

mandibular model. Int J Oral Maxillofac Implants 1995;10(3):335–44.

33. Maestre-Ferrin L, Boronat-Lopez A, Penarrocha-Diago M, et al. Augmentation procedures for deficient edentulous ridges, using onlay autologous grafts: an update. Med Oral Patol Oral Cir Bucal 2009;14(8):e402–7.

34. von Arx T, Cochran DL, Hermann JS, et al. Lateral ridge augmentation using different bone fillers and barrier membrane application. A histologic and histomorphometric pilot study in the canine mandible. Clin Oral Implants Res 2001;12(3):260–9.

35. Cardaropoli G, Araujo M, Lindhe J. Dynamics of bone tissue formation in tooth extraction sites. An experimental study in dogs. J Clin Periodontol 2003;30(9):809–18.

36. Lekovic V, Camargo PM, Klokkevold PR, et al. Preservation of alveolar bone in extraction sockets using bioabsorbable membranes. J Periodontol 1998; 69(9):1044–9.

37. Iasella JM, Greenwell H, Miller RL, et al. Ridge preservation with freeze-dried bone allograft and a collagen membrane compared to extraction alone for implant site development: a clinical and histologic study in humans. J Periodontol 2003;74(7):990–9.

38. Fiorellini JP, Howell TH, Cochran D, et al. Randomized study evaluating recombinant human bone morphogenetic protein-2 for extraction socket augmentation. J Periodontol 2005;76(4):605–13.

39. Molly L, Vandromme H, Quirynen M, et al. Bone formation following implantation of bone biomaterials into extraction sites. J Periodontol 2008;79(6): 1108–15.

40. Vance GS, Greenwell H, Miller RL, et al. Comparison of an allograft in an experimental putty carrier and a bovine-derived xenograft used in ridge preservation: a clinical and histologic study in humans. Int J Oral Maxillofac Implants 2004;19(4): 491–7.

41. Becker W, Clokie C, Sennerby L, et al. Histologic findings after implantation and evaluation of different grafting materials and titanium micro screws into extraction sockets: case reports. J Periodontol 1998;69(4):414–21.

42. Louis PJ, Gutta R, Said-Al-Naief N, et al. Reconstruction of the maxilla and mandible with particulate bone graft and titanium mesh for implant placement. J Oral Maxillofac Surg 2008;66(2): 235–45.

43. Sclar AG. Preserving alveolar ridge anatomy following tooth removal in conjunction with immediate implant placement. The Bio-Col technique. Atlas Oral Maxillofac Surg Clin North Am 1999; 7(2):39–59.

Osteoperiosteal Flaps and Local Osteotomies for Alveolar Reconstruction

Ole T. Jensen, DDS, MS[a],*, William Bell, DDS[b], Jared Cottam, DDS, MD[a]

KEYWORDS

• Osteoperiosteal flap • Osteotomy • Alveolar reconstruction

OSTEOPERIOSTEAL FLAP

The osteoperiosteal flap is a vascularized segmental osteotomy performed on alveolar bone, usually for older patients, and therefore, the effects of aging and hemodynamics must be taken into account.

Alveolar bone contains a central bone marrow and an investing tissue that includes periosteum. Blood supply to the alveolus comes from bone marrow and the periosteal tissue but there is 30% greater blood flow to the maxilla than the mandible.[1] Younger patients have a greater blood supply from the bone marrow than older patients.[2] Complete occlusion of the inferior alveolar vessels of the mandible occurs in 50% of older patients studied with angiography,[3] but this does not seem to significantly impair bone metabolism nor is it the cause of alveolar atrophy. Retrograde perfusion from the periosteal anastomosis of the facial artery seems to become more significant in aging.[4] This finding correlates with the general decrease in bone marrow blood flow caused by aging with attendant decrease in functional osteoblasts and endosteal bone-forming capacity.[5] Moreover, patients with atherosclerotic peripheral vascular disease have decreased bone blood flow that likely affects the jaw in the older patient population.[6] The blood flow to soft tissues of the periostium seems to be independent of blood flow to alveolar bone, so highly engorged gingival tissues

observed in older patients does not necessarily suggest a well-vascularized osteum.[7]

Older patients have less central and more peripheral vascularity through the outer cortex of the periosteum, therefore an osteotomy does not substantially disturb the vascular vitality from the mucoperiosteum.[8] When a bone segment is completely cut free and stripped of periosteal vascular supply, it becomes ischemic and bone cells die within 2 hours. Vascularization of the bone segment remains the sine qua non of viability for the osteoperiosteal flap.[9–13]

THE BIOLOGIC BASIS OF THE OSTEOPERIOSTEAL FLAP

The biologic basis of the osteoperiosteal flap is based on vascular studies and clinical experience with the Le Fort I osteotomy. Successful Le Fort I osteotomy depends on the preservation of adequate vascular perfusion. Careful surgical technique is necessary to maintain this perfusion. Complications associated with Le Fort I osteotomies may result from vascular ischemia resulting in the devitalization of teeth, loss of teeth, formation of periodontal defects, necrosis of gingival tissues, aseptic necrosis of entire dentoalveolar segments, and delayed union or nonunion.

Bell and colleagues[14,15] have reported primate studies that provide biologic insight into the bone healing and revascularization processes that

[a] Implant Dentistry Associates of Colorado, Oral & Maxillofacial Surgery, 8200 East Belleview Avenue, Suite 520, Greenwood Village, CO 80111, USA
[b] Department of Oral and Maxillofacial Surgery and Pharmacology, Professor Baylor College of Dentistry, Dallas, TX, USA
* Corresponding author.
E-mail address: ojensen@clearchoice.com

Oral Maxillofacial Surg Clin N Am 22 (2010) 331–346
doi:10.1016/j.coms.2010.04.003

accompany maxillary osteotomies, showing that blood flow remains sufficient after segmentation of the maxilla even with significant stretching of the vascular pedicle by up to 10 mm (**Fig. 1**). Quejada and colleagues[9] showed that a bilateral technique provides sufficient pedicles supporting a segmental maxillary osteotomy even with transection of the descending palatine vessels.[14–16] The colateral vascularity through the periosteum is sufficient even with occlusion of the major vessels.

To identify the effects of a standard circumvestibular incision, segmentation of the maxilla, stretching of the vascular pedicle, and transection of the descending palatine vessels, 4-piece Le Fort I osteotomies were performed in adult rhesus monkeys. The revascularization and bone healing associated with the procedure were studied at various intervals using microangiographic and histologic techniques. The osteotomy was made superior to the apices of all teeth except the long curvilinear canines, which were occasionally inadvertently sectioned (**Fig. 2**).

In this animal model, all soft-tissue incisions healed uneventfully.

Gingival, labial, buccal, and palatal vessels penetrated the maxillary cortical bone and anastomosed with vessels of the periodontal plexus. Dental pulps were vascularized by intraosseous dental alveolar vessels and branches from the periodontal plexi. Gingival vessels received blood from buccal mucoperiosteum and intraalveolar vessels. Soft tissues and intraosseous vessels supplied blood to the periosteum. Many vascular anastamoses interconnected the vessels of the gingival, periodontal plexi, palatal mucosa, and labiobuccal alveolar mucosa.

IMMEDIATE POSTSURGICAL SPECIMEN

Extensive areas of intraosseous ischemia were observed within all segments (**Fig. 3**A). This

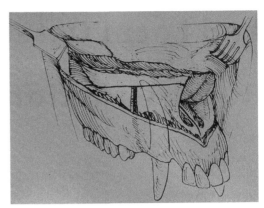

Fig. 2. Le Fort I down graft was done in a rhesus monkey to evaluate revascularization.

ischemia was particularly marked within the buccal cortex subjacent to the site of mucoperiosteal flap elevation. Although all elevated soft tissues exhibited vascularization, large avascular zones and regions of extravasated perfusant were present beneath the elevated soft-tissue flaps and between the margins of the osteotomized segments. Many of the superficial intracortical vessels beneath these zones did not contain perfusant. The distribution of the injection medium throughout the periodontal plexi and the pulps of all teeth were diminished relative to the control animal, but still present. Histologically, the avascular zones were occupied by fibrinous blood clots and inflammatory cells.

A remarkable recovery from the initial reduction of blood flow was transiently observed after surgery, clinically and experimentally (see **Fig. 3**B). Avascular anastomoses between the maxilla and its enveloping soft tissues are crucial in providing compensatory blood supply to dento-osseous segments after the nutrient medullary vascular system is transected. The vascular connections between the maxilla and its surrounding soft tissues consists of not only capillaries but also arteries and veins, which are arranged in various configurations. The multiple sources of blood supply to the maxilla and the abundant vascular communications between the hard and soft tissues constitute the biologic foundation for maintaining dento-osseous viability despite transection of the medullary blood supply after osteotomies.

ONE-WEEK SPECIMEN

At 7 days there was an increased filling of the intraosseous and periosteal vascular beds relative to the immediate postsurgical specimen (see **Fig. 3**C). The soft-tissue flaps were well vascularized but had not reattached to the underlying

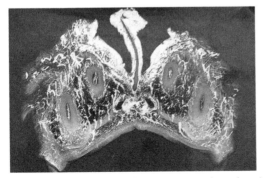

Fig. 1. Control rhesus monkey, unoperated, perfused with radio-opaque die indicating marrow and periosteal blood supply.

A

B

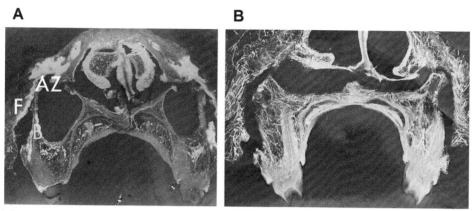

Fig. 3. (*A*) Immediately after a Le Fort I osteotomy, ischemic bone margins are evident as a result of interruption of blood flow. (*B*) Seven days postoperative Le Fort I with early revascularization as shown by radio-opaque angiography.

bone, as shown by intervening avascular areas. Although increased filling of the intraosseous circulatory bed was evident along the periphery of the osteotomy sites, direct circulation between the bone fragments had not been reestablished. Microscopic examination showed granulation tissue containing immature fibroblasts and capillary buds at the osteotomy sites and subjacent to the mucoperiosteal flaps. Many of these new capillaries were filled with injection medium. The avascular zones along the surface of the sectioned bone contained lacunae devoid of osteocytes. Within the central regions of the osteotomy sites and in some areas along the bone surface subjacent to the soft-tissue flaps, large networks of fibrin unpenetrated by capillaries persisted. Small amounts of newly formed endosteal bone extended from the margins of the osteotomized buccal bone. The periodontal space appeared normal, with micropaque-filled blood vessels of varying circumference coursing through the periodontal fibers.

Compared with the 7-day specimen, a more exuberant proliferation of vascular channels was apparent within the osteotomy sites within 2 weeks. Blood vessels from the palatal and buccal flaps in some areas had penetrated the bone to anastamose with intraosseous vessels. Numerous fine blood vessels had begun to traverse the previously avascular zones between the sectioned portions of bone. Microscopic examination of the osteotomy sites disclosed further organization of the granulation tissue. This tissue was well vascularized and contained many collagen fibers and associated fibroblasts. Within the parasagittal (palatal) osteotomy site, a small amount of newly formed bone was evident. Within the buccal osteotomy sites, the buccal periosteum was thickened, and many spicules of new bone extended

from the bony margins. New bone was also seen on the endosteal margin.

FOUR-WEEK SPECIMEN

By 4 weeks, endosteal-periosteal anastamoses had been reestablished throughout the palatal and alveolar bone (**Fig. 4**A). Numerous blood vessels from the gingival, labial, buccal, and palatal mucosa were now perfused. Intraosseous vessels frequently anastomosed with periodontal plexi. Proliferating intraosseous blood vessels restored the circulation between the sectioned bone fragments (see **Fig. 4**A). Microscopically, abundant new bone was observed within the osteotomy sites and the marrow spaces around the bone cuts (see **Fig. 4**B) contained loose fibrous connective tissue and spicules of osteoid and new bone. Empty lacunae were still present along the margins of the osteotomized segments, but many osteocytes occupied the bone away from these margins. Across the parasagittal (posterior palatal) osteotomy sites, a thick band of well-vascularized fibrous tissue was interposed between the advancing zones of new bone (**Fig. 5**A, B). Many viable osteocytes were present within the newly formed bone. Numerous small blood vessels filled with injection medium were observed within the marrow spaces. The pulp tissues of all teeth except a few of canines were perfused with micropaque. A hypervascular response (see **Fig. 5**A) was noted in the osteotomy sites where there was almost complete bony bridging between the proximal and distal segments (see **Fig. 5**B).

Vascular changes elicited by maxillary osteotomy and repositioning have been of paramount concern since the earliest surgical efforts. Several surgeons have since reported devitalization of teeth, loss of teeth and bone segments, and

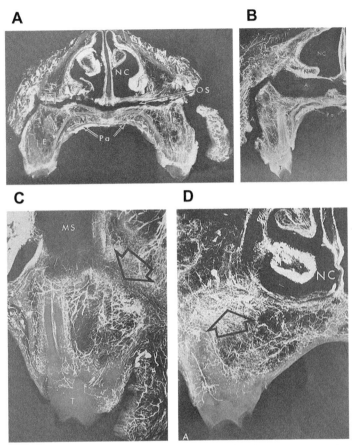

Fig. 4. (*A*) Le Fort I osteotomy healing after 1 week in a rhesus monkey demonstrates exuberant vascularity at all boney margins. (*B, C, D*) Week 2, week 4, and week 6 segmented osteotomies undergo osseous proliferation and consolidation directly related to increased vascularity.

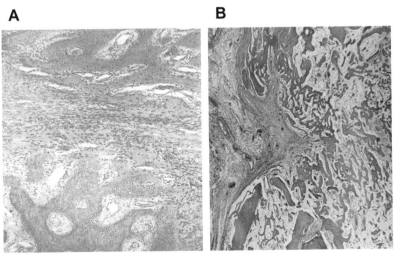

Fig. 5. (*A*) Histology of 2-week specimen indicates the fibroproliferation of early wound healing. (*B*) Later, at 6 weeks, ossification and union develops.

periodontal defects after Le Fort I osteotomies. These cases have all been attributable to maxillary hemodynamic insufficiency.

A careful assessment of the circumstances involved when small or large bone segments are lost generally shows that the operating surgeon has violated a basic biologic or surgical principle. Most frequently, the vascular pedicle has not been maintained by proper soft-tissue flap design, or circulation to the mobilized segment has not been preserved by way of attached palatal muco-periosteum. Excessively long and traumatic surgery, inappropriate selection of interdental osteotomy sites, strangulation of the circulation by imprudent use of palatal splints, and excessive stretching of the palatal mucosal pedicle are other causes of compromised wound healing.

Necrosis of an entire dentoalveolar segment after maxillary osteotomy was first reported by Parnes and Becker[17] in 1972. Incisions were performed through the interdental papillae, and full thickness mucoperiosteal flaps were reflected buccolabially and palatally so that little to no soft-tissue pedicle remained attached to the osteotomized anterior maxillary segment. This complication clearly resulted from a surgical technique that compromised the osteoperiosteal pedicle.

Of the 36 cases of aseptic necrosis after maxillary surgery reported by Lanigan and colleagues,[18] 11 cases ranged from the devitalization of teeth to the devitalization of a large dentoalveolar segment. Causes for failure included compression of the vascular pedicle with a palatal splint, improper placement of a suspension wire, excessive stripping of palatal soft tissue, overzealous use of disimpaction forceps and improper presurgical planning for patients with impaired vascular anatomy from previous maxillary surgeries.

Dodson and colleagues recently reported a prospective human cohort study that compared Le Fort I osteotomy patients in whom one group received descending palatine artery ligation, and in the other the descending palatine arteries were preserved. No significant short-term difference in the anterior maxillary gingival blood flow as measured by laser Doppler flowmetry was observed between the 2 groups.[19]

BIOLOGY OF SMALL SEGMENT WOUND HEALING

After the development of predictable, biologically based techniques for immediate repositioning of the anterior and posterior maxillary dentoalveolar segments, which usually contained between 3 and 6 teeth, the challenge remained as to whether smaller single-tooth dento-osseous segments (analogous to edentulous osteoperiosteal flaps) could be repositioned similarly. Because pedicling the segment to a relatively small amount of soft tissue could presumably imperil circulation to the mobilized dento-osseous segment, many surgeons have avoided such procedures. The biology of healing associated with the surgical repositioning of single-tooth dento-osseous segments was studied experimentally in adult mongrel dogs (**Fig. 6**).[20] Within 2 weeks after surgery, revascularization of the small dento-osseous segment was noted (**Fig. 7**).

Healing studies of nonpedicled anterior, posterior, or total maxillary osteotomies in monkeys revealed osteonecrosis, pulpal and periodontal ischemia, frank clinical infection, and exfoliating teeth. The profound clinical effects of devascularization were noted within 1 week after the experimental surgeries (**Figs. 8** and **9**).

Successful transposition of dento-osseous segments depends on preservation of viability by proper design of the soft-tissue and bony incisions. The collateral circulation within the maxilla and its enveloping soft tissues and the numerous vascular anastomoses in the maxilla permit many technical modifications of the 2 techniques used in the investigation. These early studies add further credibility to the use of small segmental osteotomy fragments of edentulous bone as long as the vascularized pedicle remains intact. Almost any combination of small dentoalveolar segments may be simultaneously mobilized and selectively repositioned to achieve the desired position.

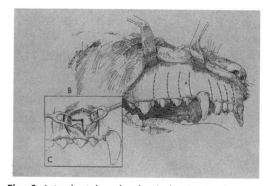

Fig. 6. Interdental and subapical osteotomies were done. Small finely tapered osteotomies were used interdentally to connect the buccal and palatal osteotomies. All the single-tooth dento-osseous segments were then fully mobilized and repositioned medially and inferiorly the width of the osteotomies. Fixation was accomplished with Erich arch bars, 24 gauge SSW, and direct bonding acrylic.

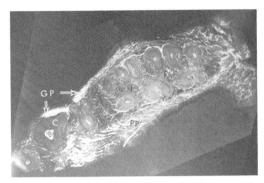

Fig. 7. A control specimen demonstrating extensive vascularity subperiostially and in the marrow space.

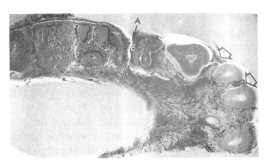

Fig. 9. Osteonecrosis from ischemia in segment left to heal for 4 weeks without pedicled blood supply.

Ultrasonic bone cutting has allowed the realization of new and safer surgical procedures. It is possible to perform multisegmental osteotomies of the palatal bone into 4 to 8 parts, which may be impossible with classic instrumentation. Consequently greater transversal displacement can be realized 10 cases had more than 10 mm of transversal displacement with stability similar to classic transverse osteotomies.[21,22]

TREATMENT PLANNING FOR THE OSTEOPERIOSTEAL FLAP

Once a surgeon is confident in the biologic basis of small segmental osteotomies and becomes familiar with the capability of the osteoperiosteal flap, there is a completely different approach to treatment planning for edentulous settings prescribed for dental implant restoration. For example, instead of tooth removal and socket bone grafting to regain lost vertical dimension, a total alveolar sandwich osteotomy may be prescribed to improve alveolar height (**Figs. 10–16**).[18] If alveolar repositioning is not done, subsequently restored implant crowns appear long and an emergence profile of the restoration may not be esthetically established even with vertical block bone grafting. Therefore, vertical alveolar problems can be treated using osteoperiosteal flaps, including sandwich osteotomies, vertical alveolar distraction osteogenesis, alveolar segmental surgery, or total jaw osteotomies when indicated.[18,19,21–23]

Treatment planning for alveolar width deficiency is similarly affected by the advent of osteoperiosteal flaps. Alveolar split bone grafts, alveolar width distraction, internal alveolar split bone grafting, and sometimes total alveolar split osteotomies (in the maxilla) are prescribed.[24–26]

THE ALVEOLAR PLANE

In the dentate state the alveolar crest around the arch can be thought of as a horizontal plane that is composed of the palatal and buccal bone height. Deviations from the alveolar plane can be found at a single bone plate, a single-tooth site, multiple tooth sites, a segmental area, or with complete alveolar deficiency. In certain settings alveolar growth with segmental hypereruption may be present.[27,28] Establishment of the right

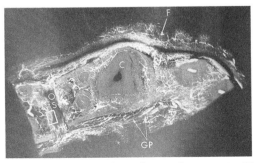

Fig. 8. Osteotomy healing of a small segment with increased vascularity noted at consolidated bone cut margins after 6 weeks healing.

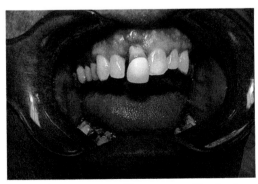

Fig. 10. The anterior maxilla presents with a fractured central incisor that has lost the facial plate and 80% of the bone on the mesial root surface of the lateral incisor.

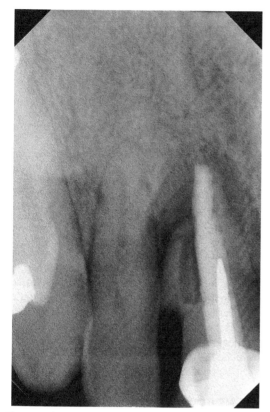

Fig. 11. The site is not conducive to socket bone grafting alone and #7 cannot be dependably preserved.

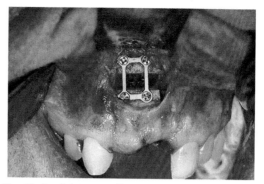

Fig. 13. By doing a small segmental sandwich osteotomy, the entire alveolar segment involving the 2 teeth is recalibrated by bringing it down about 5 mm vertically.

In partially edentulous settings of alveolar deficiency attempts should be made to recover the original alveolar plane by either vertical or lateral augmentation. In total edentulism, especially severe vertical atrophy, the use of osteotomies for grafting or distraction osteogenesis are not justified given the alternative of the fixed hybrid bridge. For the upper jaw, patients who desire a natural tooth emergence, maxillary repositioning, either by Le Fort I down graft or Le Fort I distraction, can be used.[23,29,30]

ORTHOALVEOLAR FORM

The esthetic concept of surgical recovery of orthoalveolar form, similar to orthognathic surgery, attempts to reposition osseous elements into alignment, in the case of total jaw discrepancies, into Angle Class I occlusion; and for the alveolus, into axial alignment for esthetic gingivoalveolar implant restoration. Orthoalveolar form is therefore an alveolar state in which the alveolus is at an esthetic alveolar plane, with confluent palatal and

alveolar height such that implants are placed at 1 level around the arch and bone is either augmented or removed to establish the appropriate interarch space for a restoration is desirable. In the edentulous state the restorative team can sometimes lose track of where the osseous level should best be established, so care should be taken to establish the appropriate alveolar plane based on articulated casts.

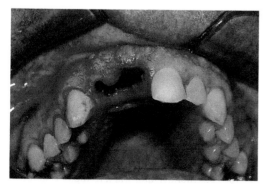

Fig. 12. Extraction of the lateral and central incisors leaves a large alveolar defect.

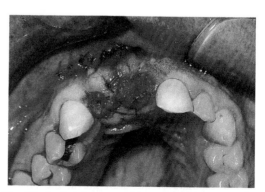

Fig. 14. Socket bone grafting proceeds with autograft/allograft and PDGF-bb with a collagen covering.

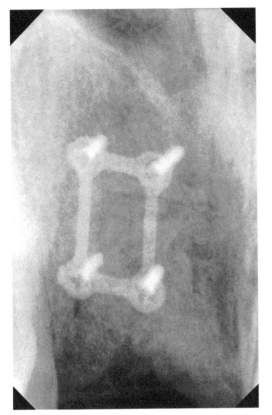

Fig. 15. The site after 4 months appears healed on periapical radiograph.

facial alveolar plates in appropriate alveolar projection to support either teeth or dental implants.[23]

ALVEOLAR PROJECTION

Alveolar projection may be thought of as the alveolar angle or alveolar tilt. The normal alveolar angle is 15° forward of the axial plane in the anterior

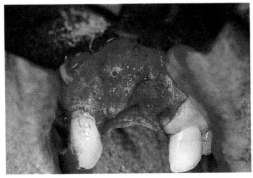

Fig. 16. Exposure of the graft site at the time of implant placement reveals a well-healed osseous site although additional minor grafting is needed.

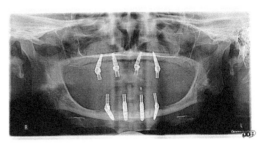

Fig. 17. The highly atrophic edentulous mandible should not be bone grafted or distracted, but instead treated by an immediate fixed restoration. Here treated with 4 implants that perforate the inferior border.

maxilla, but generally vertical posterior.[29] An alveolus can be straight vertical, forward inclined, or retro inclined. When straight or retro a ridge lap restoration is planned or a dehisced implant restoration will result. Sufficient alveolar projection is a good thing to keep in mind in trying to keep an anterior maxillary implant within bone and within the buccal line.[25]

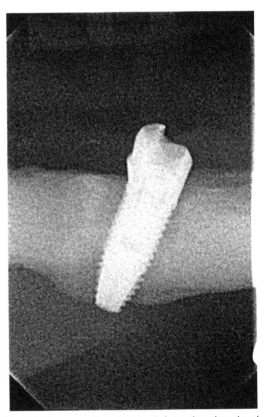

Fig. 18. Four months later the left implant has developed periosteal bone apposition at the apex of the implant.

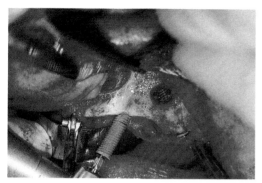

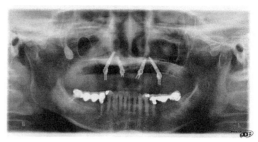

Fig. 21. This All On Four configuration is M-shaped, an angled placement technique used to avoid sinus grafting and extensive implant treatment most often done in elderly patients.

Fig. 19. The atrophic maxilla, unlike the mandible, must often rely on a grafting approach for dental implants, the exception being the M-4 All On Four technique, which gains fixation at the lateral pyriform rim above the nasal fossa.

SUBPAPILLARY BONE MORPHOLOGY

One of the key properties of the edentulous space to evaluate is the level of the bone on the adjacent teeth. An extraction of a single tooth will not result in significant papillary regression if bone height remains high around the adjacent teeth. This height of bone therefore establishes papilla height.[28,30] The presence or absence of this bone establishes criteria when an osteotomy augmentation procedure is contemplated.

When adjacent subpapillary bone is insufficient, soft-tissue augmentation may not improve papillary height. The problem must be solved by either orthodontic supereruption or osteotomy repositioning of the teeth. The first step in establishing a plan for segmental augmentation in the edentulous zone is to evaluate adjacent subpapillary bone height. When the subpapillary bone is vertically deficient, more than 4 mm, then adjacent teeth should be included in the osteotomy.[31] Orthodontic forced eruption is generally used for vertical osseous defects of 4 mm or less.[32]

TYPES OF OSTEOPERIOSTEAL FLAPS

The use of mucoperiosteal attached bone segments, particularly for edentulous bone, is seemingly unlimited. An edentulous jaw can be split, out fractured, made into island osteoperiosteal flaps, segmented, distracted, or undergo total alveolar, even full-jaw osteotomy. Small movements of 5 mm or less are often significant for alveolar reconstruction for dental implants. It seems that the key elements for a successful osteoperiosteal flap exposure are a minimal flap with little

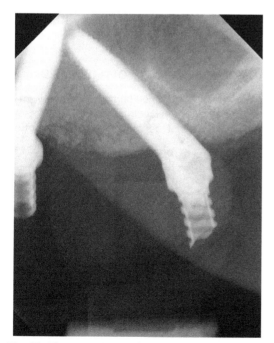

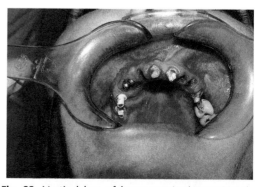

Fig. 20. The posterior implant angles anteriorly just missing the anterior sinus wall. The anterior implant angles backward just missing the lateral nasal wall.

Fig. 22. Vertical loss of bone required resetting the entire crest of the maxillary deficient bone to the alveolar plane.

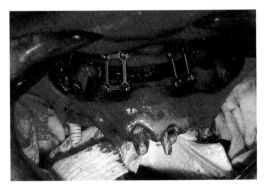

Fig. 23. Large sandwich osteotomy segments can be moved several millimeters down in conjunction with dental extractions or may include selected teeth.

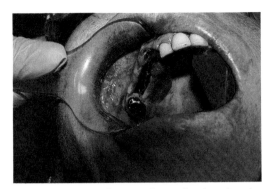

Fig. 25. Without soft-tissue flap reflection the alveolus is split using a book flap.

or no periosteal reflection, gentle osteotomy surgery including careful manipulation, and fixation to the desired position. When increased alveolar width is desired the alveolar split is done; when width and height is desired, the island osteoperiosteal flap (i-flap) may be used; when there is significant vertical loss a segmental or total jaw reposition (or distraction) is recommended.[23,30,31,33–35]

TOTAL JAW OSTEOTOMIES

Total jaw surgery for the mandible is often indicated for orthognathic deformities but seldom in preparation for implants. Most mandibular atrophy conditions, even when severe, can be treated without bone grafting using the V-4 All On Four distribution strategy (**Figs. 17** and **18**).[36] Total jaw osteotomies of the mandible for dental implant reconstruction are needed only to correct gross misalignment of the ridges.[37]

On the other hand, total jaw osteotomy such as Le Fort I down graft distraction works well for augmentation.[38] All On Four strategies graftless treatment may be helpful in highly atrophic conditions, but there is often a need for sinus floor augmentation and treatment of retro displaced maxillary position (**Figs. 19–21**).[39]

ALVEOLAR SEGMENTAL OSTEOTOMIES

One of the most common findings of edentulism is irregularity and deviation of the alveolar crest below the original dental alveolar height, often

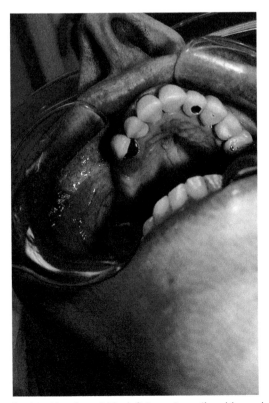

Fig. 24. Alveolar width deficiency is easily addressed with alveolar split osteotomies.

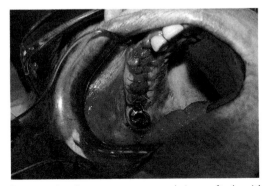

Fig. 26. The intraosseous wound is grafted with autogenous bone and covered by collagen to allow for secondary intention healing.

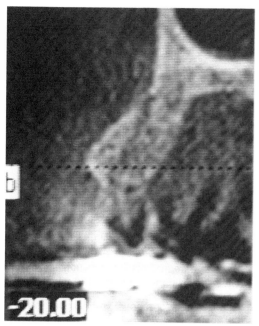

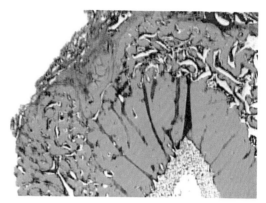

Fig. 29. The island osteoperiosteal flap grafted interpositionally in a rabbit tibia shows good consolidation of the graft and vital maintenance of the i-flap after 6 weeks healing.

Fig. 27. Four months later the alveolus presents an increased width of 5 to 6 mm.

with decreased width. When basal bone stock is adequate a segmental osteotomy can be done to relocate a segment up to the alveolar plane. The minimum effective alveolar width to do this is 4 mm at the base.[40] The regional acceleratory phenomenon (RAP) that the segment and interpositional graft undergoes during consolidation and remodeling will decrease alveolar mass an indeterminate amount.[37] When the segment is large this will not be noticeable, but very small segments mobilized with wound tension may resorb proportionately more (**Figs. 22** and **23**).

ALVEOLAR SPLIT OSTEOTOMY

Alveolar split osteotomy widens a deficient alveolus from 2 to 5 mm. This is done through a minimally reflected crestal incision. Splits can be very small, made with sequential expanding osteotomies that force bone mass buccally. This technique is excellent for gaining a few millimeters of width in deficient edentulous sites and is often used with simultaneous implant placement.[38,39,41–43] When there is excess widening, a dehiscence will be created. For moderately deficient sites a true alveolar split should be done with partial thickness dissection for wound closure or simply as a mucoperiosteal attached segment out fractured buccally, previously described as the "book flap" which is not closed primarily.[44] The book flap can gain 3 to 5 mm of width providing interosseous space for bone graft material sometimes confined by an over sewn collagen membrane. The bone segment is not fixed into place nor is the soft tissue primarily closed. This strategy is for delayed implant placement.

In highly atrophic sites, where a gain of 5 mm more is needed, distraction should be done, followed by early implant placement 5 to 6 weeks later when the distractor is removed.[37] In all of these strategies it is advisable to try and maintain

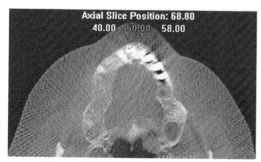

Fig. 28. Increased alveolar width helps establish an esthetic orthoalveolar form.

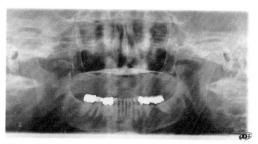

Fig. 30. An elderly patient presenting with a natural dentition, bruxism, and near complete atrophy of the maxilla.

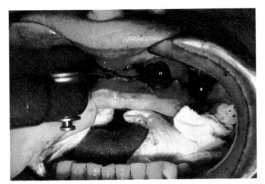

Fig. 31. A subnasal horizontal U-shaped osteotomy is performed around the arch.

2 mm of osseous facial plate thickness for the implant to be adequately covered in bone facially as thinner plates undergo replacement by creeping substitution and may resorb away (**Figs. 24–28**).[25,45]

i-FLAP OSTEOTOMIES

Island osteoperiosteal flaps (i-flap) combined with interpositional bone grafts are used to widen the arch especially in the maxilla.[35] The usefulness of the i-flap is that the facial plate can be widened and moved crestally. (Small single-tooth segments can be done, but the technique is best used segmentally.) Like all alveolar splits a 2-mm thickness of bone is desirable. Rigid fixation of the i-flap is not necessary if sufficient wound closure is obtained with late resorbing suture material. The use of bone morphogenetic protein 2 (BMP-2) may be favorable in i-flap settings especially for large segments associated with combined sinus grafting. Very thin split segments are well replaced with bone when BMP-2 is used as an interpositional graft material (**Fig. 29**).

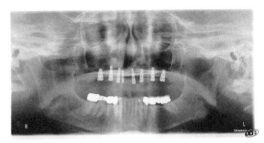

Fig. 33. After maturation, 8 implants are placed of sufficient length.

Le Fort I: Edentulous Maxilla

The Le Fort I edentulous maxillary osteotomy provides a beneficial technique to gain bone mass, reestablish vertical alveolar height, and achieve an anterior maxillary position.

The Le Fort I can be done in 1 of 3 ways

1. Sub–Le Fort I for modest vertical gain and sinus floor grafting access
2. Le Fort I distraction usually done in conjunction with sinus floor augmentation
3. Le Fort I down graft and maxillary advancement.

Sub–Le Fort I Osteotomy Down Graft

The horizontal horseshoe alveolar osteotomy of the maxilla is like an extended sandwich osteotomy, which provides increased vestibular height and increased bone mass for dental implant placement.[30] The procedure is done through a vestibular incision preserving the osseous nasal floor. The sinus membranes are first elevated and then the palate is cut transantrally around the arch. The horizontal osteotomy is made within basal bone, essentially dividing the available bone. The horseshoe need not extend to the pterygomaxillary

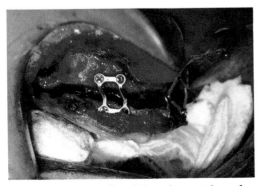

Fig. 32. The maxilla is flexed down but not down-fractured to create interosseous space to gain vertical dimension using BMP-2 for graft material.

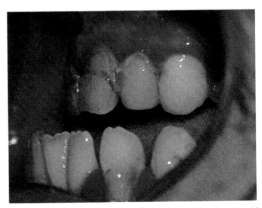

Fig. 34. A Class III jaw relationship in a patient with a condemned natural dentition caused by caries and periodontal disease.

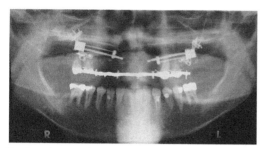

Fig. 35. The maxilla is freed with a Le Fort I and distractors are placed.

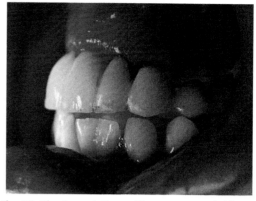

Fig. 37. The jaw relation with a temporary bridge in place following implant placement.

suture. Minimal advancement of the maxilla is possible with the vestibular approach, but if a palatal approach with a buccal pedicle is used with tunneling to make lateral cuts, the maxilla can be advanced several millimeters. The elevation of the sinus membrane and sinus grafting is not feasible with a palatal approach.

The increased bone stock in the sinus graft usually enables placement of up to 4 implants on each side for a cross-arch, splinted final restoration (**Figs. 30–33**).

Le Fort I Distraction

Distraction osteogenesis is a highly feasible outpatient procedure for the vertically deficient maxilla but sufficient alveolar bone mass for dental implants.[23] A deficiency of 10 mm horizontally and 10 mm vertically in maxillary position is usually a good indication for the distraction procedure. Distraction of the maxilla corrects interarch jaw alignment, improves alveolar cross bite tendency, provides lip support for perioral esthetics and establishes the potential for emergence profile of the restoration. For a younger female patient in the third or fourth decade this is a more natural-appearing restoration, often justifying the additional

surgical procedure in preparation for implant placement (**Figs. 34–37**).

LE FORT I DOWN GRAFT

The maxilla maxillary retrognathia and vertical deficiency can be corrected by Le Fort 1 osteotomy must be brought down and forward but the sinus membrane must first be preserved through lateral antrostomy elevation.[23] Once the maxilla is fixated into position by the use of resorbable bone plates, over grafting can be done laterally in conjunction with nasal and sinus floor grafting. This generally requires iliac bone grafting, however, BMP-2 may also be used (**Figs. 38–42**).

DISCUSSION

The use of interpositional bone grafts with various osteoperiosteal flaps is becoming more commonly used for augmentation and implant site preparation. The use of the sandwich osteotomy, in the posterior mandible, outperforms distraction osteogenesis as well as block bone grafting or guided bone regeneration.[33] Although posterior

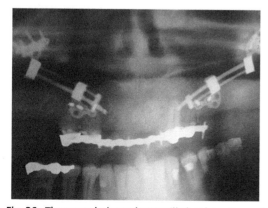

Fig. 36. Three weeks later the maxilla has been moved forward and down 12 to 15 mm.

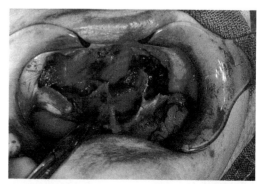

Fig. 38. A down-fractured maxilla in a 48-year-old patient with severe maxillary atrophy.

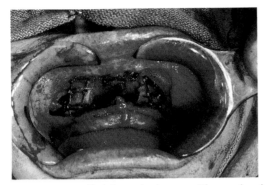

Fig. 39. The maxilla is brought down and forward and plated into position.

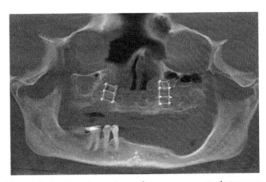

Fig. 41. Posttreatment graft on computed tomography scan.

augmentation with titanium mesh has been successful using iliac particulate graft,[46] en bloc iliac bone resorbs greater than 50%.[47] The osteotomy approach preserving a vascular pedicle often gains 8 to 10 mm; guided bone regeneration only achieves modest vertical gains.[48]

Similar results occur in the maxilla with osteoperiosteal flaps, especially for the esthetic zone. Here gingivoalveolar form is easier to obtain by a sandwich osteotomy, moving bone segments down 5 mm or more to level the alveolar plane.[18] Reconstructing and leveling the alveolar plane corrects the deformity of periodontal bone loss. This is more difficult to do with block grafting because resorption occurs in the anterior maxilla up to 40% by 1 year.[47] The sandwich approach is more stable with less resorption at the crest. The interpositional graft technique eliminates the need for vertical alveolar distraction in most cases, limiting the use of distraction to vertical movements of 10 mm or more.[31]

Full arch alveolar atrophy of the mandible and maxilla can often be treated without augmentation by using All On Four technology and/or computer-guided implant strategies. The edentulous mandible with severe atrophy can almost always be treated with a V-4 and maxilla with an M-4

technique; the letters designate implant placement angulations.[36,39] However, when the maxilla is severely or extremely resorbed, a Le Fort down graft procedure is indicated.

The Le Fort I interpositional graft procedure must be compared with an onlay grafting procedure alone. Although onlay procedures have been successful,[49] especially when combined with sinus floor grafting, the advantage of a Le Fort I down graft is maxillary repositioning into a more biomechanically advantageous implant platform. However, the onlay, onlay plus sinus floor graft, and Le Fort I interpositional graft variations have all shown favorable implant success rates when done with a delayed implant placement strategy.[49,50] The use of simultaneous implant placement combined with maxillary repositioning has also been done successfully, but requires adequate bone mass for fixation and is infrequently done.[51]

The final frontier of pedicled bone grafting, first biologically established by Bell and colleagues[14,15] nearly 50 years ago, is manipulation of a small segment of bone in preparation for dental implant

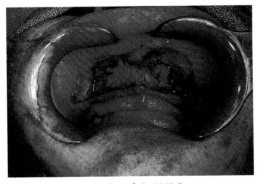

Fig. 40. Interpositional graft is BMP-2.

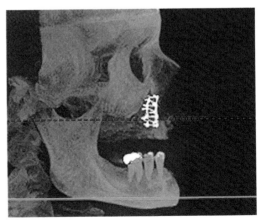

Fig. 42. Posttreatment jaw relation on computed tomography scan.

reconstruction. This is most clearly demonstrated in the alveolar split procedure where the medullary blood supply is inconsequential but the periosteal vascular pedicle is most significant to osseous healing. A rabbit tibial model determined that a thin pedicled segment separated from the tibial shaft by interpositional graft material remained vital with just periosteal blood supply.[35] However, over stripping of the bone led to ischemia and osteocyte cell death on bone margins unattached to vascular supply.[35] Another animal study compared interpositional grafting in split sites with simultaneous dental implant placement, which did not osseointegrate consistently to distracted split sites with delayed placement.[51] This indicates a reduced vascular healing capacity after medullary blood flow disruption. The buccal plate is fragile and splitting or flap reflection has been shown clinically and in animal studies to lead to complete plate resorption.[25]

The challenge for the oral and maxillofacial surgeon in dental implant site preparation is to use judgment and skill guided by biologic principles for alveolar reconstruction. Modest gains of 5 mm or less in width and height are often significant and usually extremely stable. The use of osteoperiosteal flaps should be mildly over corrected to allow for reductive remodeling.[10,52]

SUMMARY

The use of osteoperiosteal flaps provides a biologic basis to enhance alveolar implant site preparation without block grafting or guided bone regeneration. The future holds promise for the ongoing development of vascularized osteotomies for use in interpositional and distraction osteogenesis for alveolar reconstruction.

REFERENCES

1. Kaplan ML, Jeffcoat MK, Goldhaber P. Radiolabeled microsphere measurements of alveolar bone blood flow in dogs. J Periodontal Res 2006;13(4):304–8.
2. Kretschmer WB, Baciut G, Baciut M, et al. Changes in bone blood flow in segmental LeFort I osteotomies. Oral Surg Oral Med Oral Pathol Oral Radiol Endod 2009;108(2):178–83.
3. Pogrel MA, Dodson T, Tom W. Arteriographic assessment of patency of the inferior alveolar artery and its relevance to alveolar atrophy. J Oral Maxillofac Surg 1987;45(9):767–70.
4. Hellem S, Ostrup LT. Normal and retrograde blood supply to the body of the mandible in the dog. II. The role played by periosteo-medullary and symphyseal anastomoses. Int J Oral Surg 1981; 10(1):31–42.
5. Kita K, Kawai K, Hirohata K. Changes in bone marrow blood flow with aging. J Orthop Res 2005; 5(4):569–75.
6. Johnson G, Squier C. Blood flow and periodontal destruction in normal and atherosclerotic rhesus monkeys. J Periodontal Res 2006;20(5):433–43.
7. Hock JM, Kim S. Blood flow in healed and inflamed periodontal tissues of dogs. J Periodontal Res 2006; 22(1):1–5.
8. De Saint-Georges L, Miller SC. The microcirculation of bone and marrow in the diaphysis of the rat hemopoietic long bones. Anat Rec 2005;233(2):169–77.
9. Quejada JG, Kawamura H, Finn RA, et al. Wound healing associated with segmental total maxillary osteotomy. J Oral Maxillofac Surg 1986;44(5):366–77.
10. James J, Steijn-Myagkaya GL. Death of osteocytes. Electron microscopy after in vitro ischemia. J Bone Joint Surg Br 1986;68(4):620–4.
11. Berggren A, Weiland AJ, Dorfman H. The effect of prolonged ischemia time on osteocyte and osteoblast survival in composite bone grafts revascularized by microvascular anastomoses. Plast Reconstr Surg 1982;69(2):290–8.
12. Usui Y, Kawai K, Hirohata K. An electron microscopic study of the changes observed in osteocytes under ischemic conditions. J Orthop Res 1989;7(1):12–21.
13. Berggren A, Weiland AJ, Ostrup LT, et al. The effects of storage media and perfusion on osteoblast and osteocyte survival in free composite bone grafts. J Microsurg 1981;2(4):273–82.
14. Bell WH, Fonseca RJ, Kenneky JW, et al. Bone healing and revascularization after total maxillary osteotomy. J Oral Surg 1975;33(4):253–60.
15. Bell WH. Revascularization and bone healing after anterior maxillary osteotomy: a study using adult rhesus monkeys. J Oral Surg 1969;27(4):249–55.
16. You ZH, Zhang ZK, Xia JL. Blood supply of jaw bone mucoperiosteum and its role in orthognathic surgery. China J Stomatology 1991;26:31.
17. Parnes EI, Becker ML. Necrosis of the anterior maxilla following osteotomy. Oral Surg Oral Med Oral Pathol 1972;33(3):326–30.
18. Lanigan DT, Hey JH, West RA. Aseptic necrosis following maxillary osteotomies: report of 36 cases [review]. J Oral Maxillofac Surg 1990; 48(2):142–56.
19. Justus T, Chang BL, Bloomquist D, et al. Human gingival and pulpal blood flow during healing after Le Fort I osteotomy. J Oral Maxillofac Surg 2001; 59(1):2–7 [discussion: 7–8].
20. Bell WH, Schendel SA, Finn RA. Revascularization after surgical repositioning of one-tooth dentoosseous segments. J Oral Surg 1978;36:757–65.
21. Beziat JL, Bera JC, Lavandier B, et al. Ultrasonic osteotomy as a new technique in craniomaxillofacial surgery. Int J Oralmaxillofac Surg 2007;36(6): 493–500.

22. Vercellott T. Technological characteristics and clinical indications of piezoelectric bone surgery. Minerva Stomatol 2004;53(5):207–14.

23. Bell WH. Biologic basis for maxillary osteotomies. Am J Phys Anthropol 1973;38(2):279–89.

24. Jensen OT, Kuhlke L, Bedard JF, et al. Alveolar segmental sandwich osteotomy for anterior maxillary vertical augmentation prior to implant placement. J Oral Maxillofac Surg 2006;64(2):290–6 [erratum in J Oral Maxillofac Surg 2006;64(6):997].

25. Jensen OT, Leopardi A, Gallegos L. The case for bone graft reconstruction including sinus grafting and distraction osteogenesis for the atrophic edentulous maxilla. J Oral Maxillofac Surg 2004;62(11):1423–8.

26. Jensen OT, Block M. Alveolar modification by distraction osteogenesis. Atlas Oral Maxillofac Surg Clin North Am 2008;16(2):185–214.

27. Robiony M, Costa F, Politi M. Alveolar sandwich osteotomy of the anterior maxilla. J Oral Maxillofac Surg 2006;64(9):1453–4.

28. Oda T, Suzuki H, Yokota M, et al. Horizontal alveolar distraction of the narrow maxillary ridge for implant placement. J Oral Maxillofac Surg 2004;62(12):1530–4.

29. Laster Z, Rachmiel A, Jensen OT. Alveolar width distraction osteogenesis for early implant placement. J Oral Maxillofac Surg 2005;63(12):1724–30.

30. Jensen OT, Ellis E III, Glick P. Book bone flap. In: Jensen OT, editor. The osteoperiosteal flap. Chicago: Quintessence Pub; 2010. p. 87–100. Chapter 6.

31. Muñoz-Guerra MF, Naval-Gías L, Capote-Moreno A. Le Fort I osteotomy, bilateral sinus lift, and inlay bone-grafting for reconstruction in the severely atrophic maxilla: a new vision of the sandwich technique, using bone scrapers and piezosurgery. J Oral Maxillofac Surg 2009;67(3):613–8.

32. Gössweiner S, Watzinger F, Ackerman KL, et al. Horseshoe Le Fort I osteotomy: an augmentation technique for the severely atrophied maxilla–an eight-year follow-up. J Long Term Eff Med Implants 1999;9(3):193–202.

33. Jensen OT, Cockrell R, Kuhlke L, et al. Anterior maxillary alveolar distraction osteogenesis: a prospective 5-year clinical study. Int J Oral Maxillofac Implants 2002;17(1):52–68.

34. Jensen OT. Alveolar segmental "sandwich" osteotomies for posterior edentulous mandibular sites for dental implants. J Oral Maxillofac Surg 2006;64(3):471–5.

35. Allen F, Smith DG. An assessment of the accuracy of ridge-mapping in planning implant therapy for the anterior maxilla. Clin Oral Implants Res 2000;11(1):34–8.

36. Spielman HP. Influence of the implant position on the aesthetics of the restoration. Pract Periodontics Aesthet Dent 1996;8(9):897–904.

37. Ryser MR, Block MS, Mercante DE. Correlation of papilla to crestal bone levels around single tooth implants in immediate or delayed crown protocols. J Oral Maxillofac Surg 2005;63(8):1184–95.

38. Chang LC. Effect of bone crest to contact point distance on central papilla height using embrasure morphologies. Quintessence Int 2009;40(6):507–13.

39. Chang LC. The association between embrasure morphology and central papilla recession: a noninvasive assessment method. Chang Gung Med J 2007;30(5):445–52.

40. Brindis MA, Block MS. Orthodontic tooth extrusion to enhance soft tissue implant esthetics. J Oral Maxillofac Surg 2009;67(11 Suppl):49–59.

41. Raghoebar GM, Stellingsma K, Meijer HJ, et al. Vertical distraction of the severely resorbed edentulous mandible: an assessment of treatment outcome. Int J Oral Maxillofac Implants 2008;23(2):299–307.

42. Jensen OT, Mogyoros R, Alterman M, et al. Island osteoperiosteal flap. In: Jensen OT, editor. The osteoperiosteal flap. Chicago: Quintessence Pub; 2010. Chapter 7.

43. Jensen OT, Cullum DR, Baer D. Marginal bone stability using 3 different flap approaches for alveolar split expansion for dental implants: a 1-year clinical study. J Oral Maxillofac Surg 2009;67(9):1921–30.

44. Reyneke JP, Evans WG. Surgical manipulation of the occlusal plane. Int J Adult Orthodon Orthognath Surg 1990;5(2):99–110.

45. Pelo S, Gasparini G, Moro A, et al. Segmental Le Fort I osteotomy with bone grafting in unilateral severely atrophied maxilla. Int J Oral Maxillofac Surg 2009;38(3):246–9.

46. Jensen OT, Adams MW. All on 4 treatment of highly atrophic mandible with mandibular V-4: report of 2 cases. J Oral Maxillofac Surg 2009;67(7):1503–9.

47. Chiapasco M, Casentini P, Zaniboni M. Bone augmentation procedures in implant dentistry. Int J Oral Maxillofac Implants 2009;24(Suppl):237–59.

48. Jensen OT, Adams MW. The maxillary M-r: a technical and biomechanical note for all on 4 management of severe maxillary atrophy—report of 3 cases. J Oral Maxillofac Surg 2009;67(8):1739–44.

49. Jensen OT. Sandwich osteotomy bone graft in the anterior mandible. In: Jensen OT, editor. The osteoperiosteal flap. Chicago: Quintessence Pub; 2010. Chapter 11.

50. Shih MS, Norrdin RW. Regional acceleration of remodeling during healing of bone defects in beagles of various ages. Bone 1985;6(5):377–9.

51. Blus C, Szmukler-Moncler S. Split-crest and immediate implant placement with ultra-sonic bone surgery: a 3-year life-table analysis with 230 treated sites. Clin Oral Implants Res 2006;17(6):700–7.

52. Weingart D, Joos U, Hurzeler MB, et al. Restoration of maxillary residual ridge atrophy using LeFort I osteotomy with simultaneous endosseous implant placement: technical report. Int J Oral Maxillofac Implants 1992;7(4):529–35.

Bone Materials Available for Alveolar Grafting

Joseph Deatherage, DMD, MD

KEYWORDS

- Alveolar graft • Bone graft • Bone materials • Bony defects

Large numbers of bone grafting procedures are performed in the United States annually. Cost estimates for these bone grafting procedures exceed $2.5 billion.[1] Autografts or allograft materials are used for most often for these procedures. The current gold standard is the autologous bone graft because it consistently yields the best results. Patients' own bone is a living cellular transfer of tissue and the only disadvantage is the donor site. Common sites for harvesting autografts include intraoral sites, such as ramus or chin bone. Other distant sites include iliac crest, tibia, and cranial bone. The anterior iliac crest provides abundant cancellous bone and is ideal for condensing into bony defects, such as alveolar cleft. Unfortunately, cancellous bone does not remain stable as an onlay or subperiosteal bone graft for reconstruction of the atrophic maxilla or mandible. Cortical bone, such as cranial struts, or mandibular block grafts do increase width and height when rigidly fixated. Autografts have multiple qualities that make them ideal for bone grafting in preparation for dental implants. These desirable properties stem primarily from the fact that autografts are cellular, osteoconductive, osteogenic, and osteoinductive. These properties predictably result in new bone growth. The principles of bone grafting are not new to oral and maxillofacial surgeons but the result must be predictable in smaller locations often compromised by adjacent dentition.

There is a long history of using bone grafting techniques to restore craniofacial bony defects (**Fig. 1**). An early example of bone grafting occurred in 1668. In this case a Dutch surgeon, Job van Meekeren, repaired a cranial defect in a soldier with a piece of dog skull. This graft was later removed some years later for religious reasons.

Fred Albee, MD, was a pioneer in developing early autologous bone grafting techniques. He developed an early bone mill for graft preparation. Much of his work was performed on soldiers with orthopedic injuries sustained in World War I. Oral and maxillofacial surgeons, including Auxhausen, Boyne, and Marx, have also established bone grafting protocols for oral reconstruction.

A major advance in bone grafting possibilities occurred with the discovery of bone morphogenic protein (BMP), reported by Marshall Urist,[2] MD, in 1965 (**Fig. 2**). Since that initial report, at least 20 BMPs have been identified as part of larger family of transforming growth factor β. The essence of this area of grafting is that contained within the extracellular matrix of bone are proteins, which can be isolated. These proteins stimulate the formation of new bone. BMP from recombinant sources is now available as an off-the-shelf material for bone grafting. BMP is delivered by a collagen carrier.

Harvesting autologous bone grafts is associated with significant morbidity related to the donor surgical site. Complications associated with donor sites include pain, which can exceed the pain associated with original surgical site. Infections, hematoma, seroma, and gait disturbance, although infrequent, are a significant source of

Department of Oral and Maxillofacial Surgery, University of Alabama at Birmingham, 1530 Third Avenue South, SDB 419, Birmingham, AL 35294-0007, USA
E-mail address: jrddmdmd@msn.com

Oral Maxillofacial Surg Clin N Am 22 (2010) 347–352
doi:10.1016/j.coms.2010.06.003
1042-3699/10/$ – see front matter © 2010 Published by Elsevier Inc.

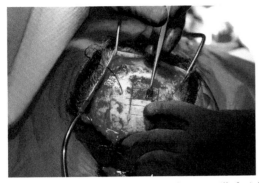

Fig. 1. Cranial bone grafting for maxillofacial reconstruction.

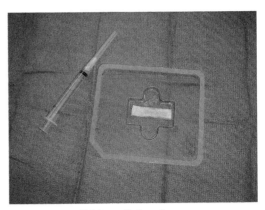

Fig. 2. BMP available as "Infuse."

morbidity. The amount of bone available for harvest is limited, especially from local sites, such as the chin or ramus.

As a result of the shortcomings associated with harvesting autologous bone, many substitute materials have been developed. (**Tables 1** and **2**; **Box 1**) Allograft and xenograft are now available as freeze-dried banked bone and commonly used for reconstituting bony defects or extending limited autografts (**Fig. 3**). These materials are harvested from cadavers and bovine sources. Allograft/xenograft materials eliminate the shortcomings of a donor site and simplify the reconstruction so that many procedures can be done in a dental office. The bone is typically treated by freezing, freeze-drying, irradiation, and other manipulations to render the material free of contamination. Fresh frozen bone is harvested and washed. It is then stored in quarantine at $-80°C$ for 6 months. This process helps eliminate

any potential source of infection and the biologically active proteins are preserved.[3]

Other techniques use ethylene oxide and/or irradiation to reduce the risk of disease transmission. Nonetheless, the risk of disease transmission is not zero. It has been estimated that the risk of HIV transmission associated with allograft bone is 1 case out of 1.6 million.[4] Other infectious agents, such as hepatitis B and C, are associated with allograft material.[5]

Rigorous screening of donors has reduced the risk of disease transmission associated with osseous allografts. Other types of infection associated with allografts have been reported. One patient who underwent reconstructive orthopedic surgery died from an infection caused by *Clostridium sordellii*. This infection generated a Centers for Disease Control and Prevention investigation, which detected 25 other cases of allograft-induced infection.[6] In summary, donor screening

Table 1		
Bone substitute synopsis		
Graft Material	**Characteristics**	**Examples**
Allograft	A graft that is taken from a member of the same species as the host but is genetically dissimilar	Cadaver cortical/cancellous bone, FDBA, DFDBA
Xenograft	Grafts derived from a genetically different species than the host	Bio-Oss, coralline HA, red algae
Alloplast (synthetic materials)	Fabricated graft materials	Calcium sulfate, bioactive glasses, HA, NiTi

Abbreviations: DFDBA, decalcified freeze-dried bone allograft; FDBA, freeze-dried bone allograft; HA, hydroxyapatite; NiTi, porous nickel titanium.

From Kao ST, Scott DD. A review of bone substitutes. Oral Maxillofacial Surg Clin North Am 2007;19:513–21; with permission.

Table 2
Bone graft material characteristics

Characteristic	Graft Material
Osteogenesis	Autograft
Osteoinduction	BMP
	DFDBA
	DBM
Osteoconduction	Bio-Oss
	Calcium phosphates
	Calcium sulfate
	Collagen
	FDBA
	Glass ionomers
	HA
	NiTi

Abbreviations: DBM, demineralized bone matrix; DFDBA, decalcified freeze-dried bone allograft; FDBA, freeze-dried bone allograft; HA, hydroxyapatite; NiTi, porous nickel titanium.

From Kao S, Scott DD. A review of bone substitutes. Oral Maxillofacial Surg Clin North Am 2007;19:513–21; with permission.

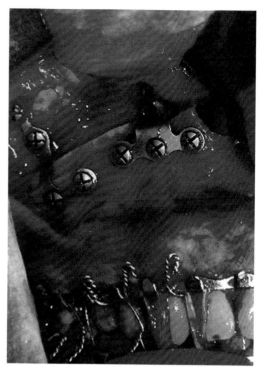

Fig. 3. Freeze-dried tibial bone is rehydrated and cut to fit between the lateral wall of maxilla in large advancements of the maxilla in surgical treatment of obstructive sleep apnea. (*Courtesy of* Dr Peter Waite, Birmingham, AL.)

and tissue processing reduces the risk of disease transmission. Sterilization techniques, however, destroy the cellular and osteoinductive properties of the graft material.

In view of these considerations, the shortcomings associated with autologous and allogeneic bone grafting have stimulated the search for alternative materials and techniques.

Allograft-based materials contain the biologically active proteins found in the extracellular matrix of bone. These biologically active proteins contain many factors, such as BMP, as described in the article elsewhere in this issue. They may also contain other agents involved in stimulating the formation of new bone. Other forms of allograft

bone include freeze-dried bone (**Fig. 4**). Freeze-dried bone can be further divided into mineralized and demineralized forms (**Fig. 5**).

Preparation of demineralized bone graft involves processing the bone with hydrochloric acid, which makes these proteins available to stimulate new bone formation. There is some evidence that freeze-drying diminishes the amount of osteoinduction and new bone formation in comparison to autologous bone and, therefore, diminished bone strength.[7] There are many commercial sources of this type of graft material. Allografts and xenografts are valuable contributors to autografts as extenders or fillers for contour defects (**Figs. 6** and **7**). A good example of this is combining demineralized freeze-dried bone over autologous block grafts, which may act as a protective membrane.

Ceramic-based materials constitute a large percentage of materials available for restoring bony defects. This material can be used alone or together with other substances to fill bony defects. These products clinically work well in sinus lifting as a bone graft extender.

Box 1
Bone graft classification

1. Allograft-based materials: cadaver, freeze-dried bone allograft, and decalcified freeze-dried bone.
2. Ceramic-based materials: calcium sulfate, calcium phosphates, bioactive glass, and hydroxyapatite.
3. Factor-based materials: platelet-rich plasma, BMP, and other inductive proteins.
4. Cell-based materials: autogenous living vital bone, cell cultures, and stem cell regeneration.

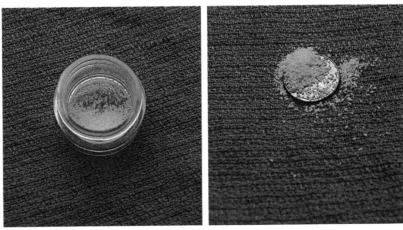

Fig. 4. Freeze-dried allograft (Oragraft). (*From* LifeNet Health, Virginia Beach, VA; with permission.)

The rationale used to support the use of ceramic materials is that they mimic the inorganic component of bone and allow new bone with connective tissue to form a bone matrix. Specific examples of ceramics include calcium sulfate (plaster of Paris), calcium phosphates, bioactive glasses, inorganic component of bovine bone, and hydroxyapatite.

There are several shortcomings associated with these materials, including brittleness, and they are not appropriate for load-bearing applications. Also, they are at best osteoconductive. They are not osteoinductive and do not stimulate new bone formation.

This type of material works best for filling contour defects. It may also be used with some efficacy to extend the volume of more biologically active materials, such as allogenic bone. Ceramics offer a poor substitute for viable bone in the support of dental implants. It they become contaminated as in peri-implantitis, this can result in rapid loss of osseointegration and implant failure.

Factor-based bone graft materials represent a viable option for restoration of bony defects. Chief among these are those that contain BMP in a collagen delivery vehicle (**Fig. 8**). This type of material stimulates new bone formation by inducing undifferentiated mesenchymal cells to migrate into the graft material and transform into living vital bone.

In March 2007, Infuse Bone Graft was approved by the Food and Drug Administration for sinus augmentation and localized alveolar ridge bony defects. In a study that investigated the use of this material, significant amounts of living host bone were developed.[8]

In native bone, miniscule amounts of BMP and other growth factors necessary for bony healing are sequestered in the mineralized matrix. These biologically active proteins are activated during bony fracture, which exposes them to the cellular environment. This in turn results in fracture healing. Chief among these growth factors, BMP induces the migration of undifferentiated, pluripotent mesenchymal cells. These cells undergo differentiation to chondroblasts, which ultimately results in new bone formation through endochondral ossification. This type of graft when used to

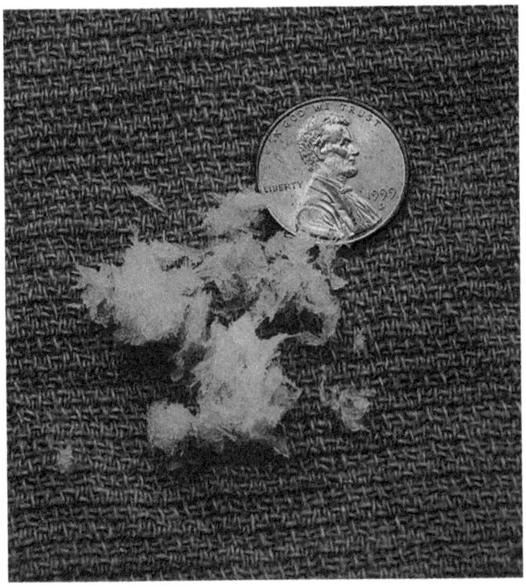

Fig. 5. Grafton: a demineralized bone matrix. (*From* Osteotech, Eatontown, NJ; with permission.)

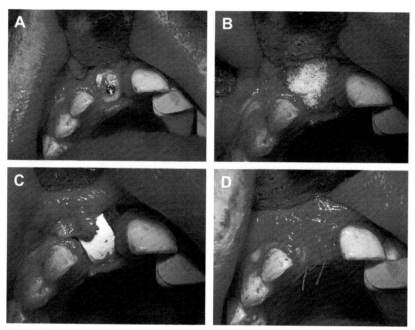

Fig. 6. (*A*) Block graft secured into alveolar defect, (*B*) block covered with demineralized freeze-dried bone, (*C*) collagen membrane, (*D*) soft tissue flap advancement.

restore alveolar defects results in vital bone. Shortcomings of this material are chiefly related to the cost of the material.

The future of bone grafting will likely use cell-based materials. Currently, technology exists to stimulate undifferentiated stem cells in vitro to develop into osteogenic lines. Various growth factors can be added to cell media to transform these cells into bone forming osteoblasts.

These cells can then be added to ceramic scaffolds to produce bone like structures to fill bony defects.

In conclusion, the restoration of bony defects has followed an interesting course through history. From the early use of animal materials to bone grown in the laboratory, the goal of restoring bony defects has generated ingenuity in solving these significant clinical challenges.

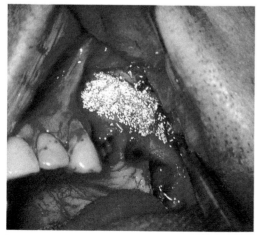

Fig. 7. Osteograf: a xenograft of natural hydroxyapatite.

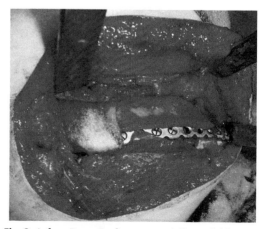

Fig. 8. Infuse Bone Graft: commercially available BMP.

REFERENCES

1. Giannoudis PV, Dinopoulos H, Tsiridis E. Bone substitutes: an update. Injury 2005;36(Suppl 3):S20–7.
2. Urist MR. Bone formation by autoinduction. Science 1965;150(698):893–9.
3. Simpson D, Kakarala G, Hampson, et al. Viable cells survive in fresh frozen bone allografts. Acta Orthop 2007;78:26.
4. Boyce T, Edwards J, Scarborough N. Allograft bone. The influence of processing on safety and performance. Orthop Clin North Am 1999;30(4):571–81.
5. Conrad E, Gretch D, Obermeyer K, et al. Transmission of the hepatitis-C virus by tissue transplantation. J Bone Joint Surg Am 1995; 77(2):214–24.
6. Centers for Disease Control and Prevention. Update: allograft-associated bacterial infections – United States, 2002. MMWR Morb Mortal Wkly Rep 2002; 51(10):207–10.
7. Gazdag A, Lane J, Glaser D, et al. Alternative to autogenous bone graft: efficacy and indications. J Am Acad Orthop Surg 1995;3:1.
8. Boyne P, Marx R, Triplett G, et al. A feasibility study evaluating rh BMP2/absorbable collagen sponge for maxillary sinus floor augmentation. Int J Periodontics Restorative Dent 1997;17(1): 11–25.

Vertical Ridge Augmentation Using Titanium Mesh

Patrick J. Louis, DDS, MD

KEYWORDS

- Vertical ridge augmentation
- Titanium mesh • Reconstruction

According to the US Department of Health and Human Services, *Oral Health in America: A Report of the Surgeon General* released in 2000, the prevalence of edentulism in individuals 65 years of age or greater is 33.1%.[1]

With tooth loss, there is increased bone loss of the alveolus.[2,3] In some cases alveolar bone loss can be severe. Severe bone loss may cause difficulty for patients wearing a conventional prosthesis or being restored with dental implants. Severe alveolar bone loss can result in malnutrition, poor self-esteem, multiple dental visits for failed prosthesis, and jaw fracture (**Fig. 1**).[4] In many cases, patients with loss of alveolar bone height or width may require reconstructive procedures.

Vertical ridge augmentation remains a challenge in the reconstruction of the atrophic maxilla and mandible. The main problem arises from the need to expand the soft-tissue envelope and achieve the proper bony architecture. Techniques that have been developed to solve or circumvent this problem include onlay bone grafting with particulate bone graft, block bone graft, barrier techniques with permanent or resorbable membranes, distraction osteogenesis, vascularized ridge splitting techniques, sinus lifts, nerve repositioning techniques, short implants, and angled implants. All of these techniques have advantages and disadvantages.[5–23] This article focuses on augmentation procedures using titanium mesh, which acts as a barrier and physical support of the soft tissue over the bone graft.

BACKGROUND

In 1973, Gargiulo and colleagues[24] published an article entitled *Use of titanium mesh in autogenous bone marrow repair of non-united mandibular fracture*. In 1983, Dr Gregory Cobetto and colleagues[25] reported on the treatment of 120 patients with mandibular fractures using malleable titanium mesh plates (**Fig. 2**). Titanium has been used in multiple applications and, more recently, as a barrier membrane for alveolar ridge augmentation.[20,26–30]

The use of titanium mesh for reconstruction of the atrophic alveolus was first introduced by Dr Philip Boyne in 1985.[26] In his article, he reported on the technique for osseous restoration of deficient edentulous maxillary ridges in 15 patients who were followed from 3 to 10 years. He described a technique using titanium mesh, which he contoured over edentulous dental models that had been restored to a more ideal ridge form. This custom-contoured mesh was sterilized and used to contain the bone graft at the time of surgery (**Fig. 3**). Resorption of 10% to 20% was reported in this patient group. This technique was designed to reduce ridge resorption after bone grafting without a barrier membrane, which had been shown to have 70% resorption after 6 years.[31]

Although several membranes have been introduced and used as a barrier, titanium seems to have some distinct advantages (**Table 1**). With the use of barrier membranes, it has been shown that bone can be regenerated beyond the skeletal

Residency Program, Department of Oral and Maxillofacial Surgery, University of Alabama at Birmingham, SDB 419, 1919 7th Avenue South, Birmingham, AL 35294-0007, USA
E-mail address: plouis@uab.edu

Oral Maxillofacial Surg Clin N Am 22 (2010) 353–368
doi:10.1016/j.coms.2010.04.005
1042-3699/10/$ – see front matter © 2010 Published by Elsevier Inc.

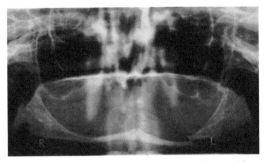

Fig. 1. Spontaneous fracture in a patient with a severely atrophic mandible.

envelope.[32–34] Rasmusson and colleagues,[35] in a simple laboratory animal model, observed that when a barrier membranes is present throughout the healing phase of a bone graft, little or no bone resorption occurred compared with membranes removed during the healing phase. If the membrane was removed early in the healing phase, there was loss of bone similar to grafts with no membrane (**Fig. 4**).

TECHNIQUE
Management of the Edentulous Maxilla

In the augmentation technique the desired ridge height is determined using a surgical guide and three-dimensional imaging. Once the desired

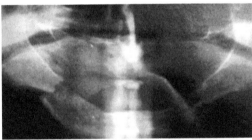

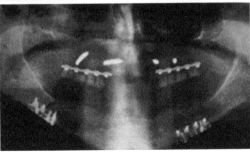

Fig. 2. Early use of titanium mesh for the management of mandibular fractures. (*Adapted from* Cobetto GA, McClary SA, Zallen RD. Treatment of mandibular fractures with malleable titanium mesh plates: a review of 120 cases. J Oral Maxillofac Surg 1983;41(9):597–600; with permission).

vertical augmentation is determined, the surgical procedure is as follows.

An incision is made approximately 5 mm below the depth of the maxillary vestibule extending posterior. A subperiosteal dissection is developed to expose the maxillary ridge and the hard palate. The greater palatine neurovascular bundle is preserved and is the posterior extent of the dissection on the hard palate. The lateral and anterior aspect of the maxilla and the tuberosity are completely exposed. The superior extent of the dissection is just below the infraorbital nerve. An osteotomy is created along the lateral wall of the maxillary sinus to perform a simultaneous sinus lift. The superior extent of the maxillary sinus window should be kept to a minimum because the bone superior to the window is desirable for fixation of the titanium mesh. Once the sinus membrane elevation is complete, the precontoured titanium mesh is chosen based on the desired augmentation. Osteomed (Osteomed Corp, Addison, TX, USA) currently provides 2 sizes of hemi trays and 2 sizes of anterior trays for augmentation (**Fig. 5**).

When large vertical heights are planned, the larger tray is usually indicated. For augmentation of the entire ridge, 2 hemi trays are used. These trays can be trimmed to create space for the nasal passage and extend superior to the sinus window but below the infraorbital nerve. It is important when contouring the mesh to eliminate sharp edges. Any contoured or cut sections of the mesh should be bent so that it extends toward the bone. Once the contouring of the tray is complete and the fit is satisfactory, the augmentation of the maxillary sinus floor is completed first. After a satisfactory fill of the sinus floor is achieved, the titanium mesh trays are filled with the bone graft material. Once the trays have been filled with bone graft material, they are placed into position and secured with at least 2 screws along the facial aspect of the maxilla and 1 screw along the midline of the palate. Once the trays have been secured into position, the wound can be closed. It is recommended that the wound be closed in layers with a deep closure using 3.0 resorbable suture such as Vicryl (Ethicon Inc, Somerville, NJ, USA) and the mucosa can then be closed with a long-lasting resorbable suture as well such as 4–0 Monocryl (Ethicon Inc, Somerville, NJ, USA) or Vicryl (**Figs. 6** and **7**).

Management of the Partially Edentulous Maxilla

When augmenting the partially edentulous maxilla, modification of the technique described earlier can

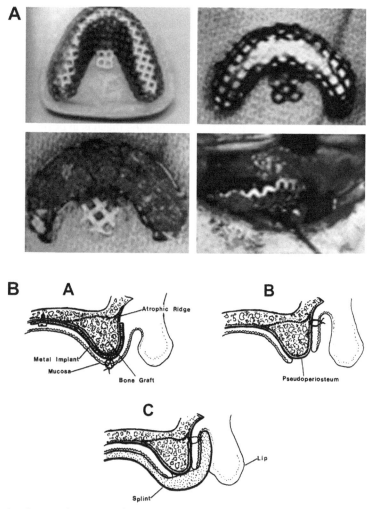

Fig. 3. (*A*) Custom titanium mesh contoured and packed with bone graft. (*B*) Diagram of the ridge augmentation and vestibuloplasty described by Dr Boyne. (*Adapted from* Boyne PJ, Cole MD, Stringer D, et al. A technique for osseous restoration of deficient edentulous maxillary ridges. J Oral Maxillofac Surg 1985;43(2):87–91; with permission).

Table 1
Advantages and disadvantages of precontoured titanium mesh

Advantages	Disadvantages
Height augmentation	Cost
Width augmentation	High rate of exposure
Ideal shape	Additional contouring
Biocompatible	needed
Rigid	
Vestibuloplasty at time of mesh removal	

be used. A crestal or vestibular incision can be used for exposure of the ridge. When a crestal incision is used, a releasing incision is often required at least 1 to 2 teeth on either side of the defect. When a vestibular approach is used an incision is made lateral to the depth of the maxillary vestibule. The incision should be curved toward the line angle of the tooth next to the defect. Care should be taken to stop the incision near the junction of the attached mucosa. The subperiosteal dissection is performed, tunneling into the crest of the ridge as well as onto the palatal surface through this incision. The mucosa is mobilized around the tooth next to the defect on either side. Care must be taken to avoid tearing of the gingival cuff. Once the mucosa is mobilized, the desired contoured mesh can be chosen. When using the precontoured mesh, the material must be cut to the

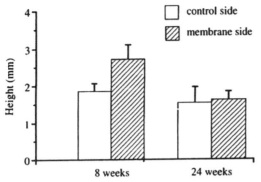

Fig. 4. Mean bone graft heights in the rabbit tibia when covered with a membrane versus a control side with no membrane at 8 weeks. Bone graft heights at 24 weeks after the membranes were removed at 8 weeks and allowed to heal for an additional 16 weeks. Note the amount of resorption begins to equal that of the control side. (*Adapted from* Rasmusson L, Meredith N, Kahnberg KE, et al. Effects of barrier membranes on bone resorption and implant stability in onlay bone grafts. An experimental study. Clin Oral Implants Res 1999;10(4): 267–77; with permission).

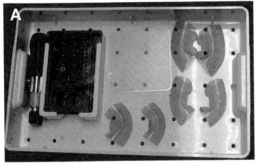

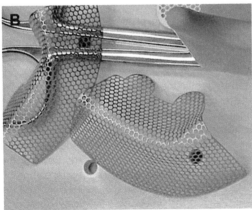

Fig. 5. Titanium mesh preformed trays. (*A*) OsteoMed kit showing trays available in various sizes, screw drive, and screws. (*B*) Close-up of a hemi-arch tray from the OsteoMed system.

desired length. It is then tied into position and contoured accordingly. Once the mesh is contoured the tray can be filled with the desired bone graft material. Cortical perforations of the bone are not necessary. If the clinician chooses to perforate the bone, the planned position of the retaining screw for the mesh must be considered so as not to create any perforations in this location. Once the mesh is in position, it is secured with at least 2 screws on the facial surface. The soft tissue can now be closed. When a crestal incision is used for exposure, the periosteum must be released along the facial vestibule to facilitate a tension-free closure of the wound. This is usually not necessary when a vestibular incision is used. The incision can be closed in layers as described earlier (**Fig. 8**).

Management of Edentulous Atrophic Mandible

When augmenting the atrophic edentulous mandible, an intraoral or extraoral approach can be used. The intraoral approach is more straightforward. In this technique an incision is made in the depth of the mandibular vestibule just anterior to the retromolar pad extending anteriorly across the midline. A subperiosteal dissection is achieved. Care must be taken to identify and protect the mental nerves. In the extremely atrophic mandible, the inferior alveolar nerve may be exposed along the crest as a result of dehiscence of the canal. A preferred technique is to start anteriorly and identify the mental foramina and then dissect posteriorly over the crest. With this technique the dissection is carried onto the lingual surface of the mandible in a subperiosteal fashion. The lingual extent of the dissection anteriorly is to the genial tubercles. The genioglossus and geniohyoid should not be detached. Once the mandible is exposed the 2 hemi trays are chosen based on the desired level of augmentation. This is determined by preoperative planning with study models and radiographs. The mesh is contoured and trimmed to fit. Relief over the mental foramina is necessary to avoid injury to the nerve. It is desirable to extend the mesh to the posterior aspect of the mandible in the region of the retromolar pad as the crest of the ridge begins to turn superiorly to form the ramus. This procedure is done to avoid any sharp areas at the end of the mesh that may later become exposed. In patients with larger mandibles, 2 trays may not be long enough to extend posteriorly to the retromolar region and cover the anterior aspect of the mandible. In these cases, a third piece of mesh must be contoured and overlapped onto the anterior aspects of both

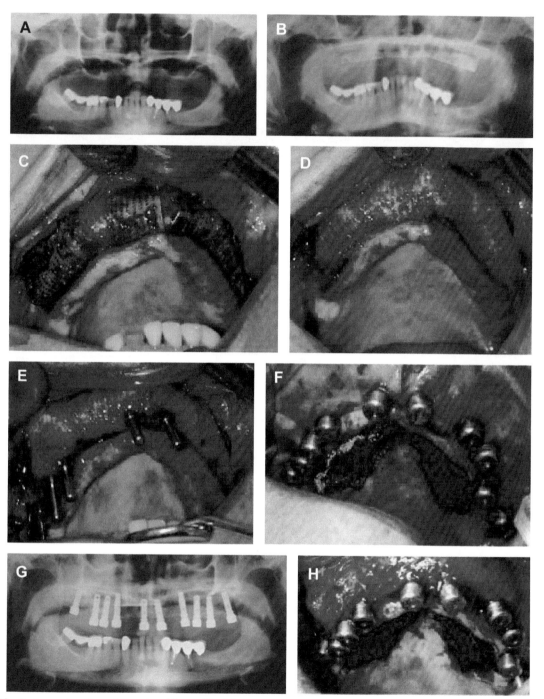

Fig. 6. Reconstruction of the atrophic maxilla. (*A*) Preoperative radiograph showing an atrophic maxillary ridge. (*B*) Postoperative radiograph with titanium mesh in place. (*C*) Maxillary ridge at the time of uncovering of the mesh at 8 months after placement. (*D*) Maxillary ridge after mesh removal. Note the pseudoperiosteum overlying the ridge. (*E*) Maxillary ridge with paralleling pins in place. (*F*) Maxillary ridge after the implants have been uncovered. Note the absence of attached gingiva around the implants and the shallow vestibule. Grafts have been harvested from the palate and surgical dressings are in place. (*G*) Postoperative radiograph after implants have been uncovered and healing caps are in place. (*H*) Maxillary ridge after a supraperiosteal dissection has been preformed. (*I*) Maxillary ridge with meshed palatal grafts in place. (*J*) Maxillary ridge after healing of the palatal graft. Note the amount of keratinized tissue around the implants. (*K*) Frontal view of the maxillary ridge reconstructed with fixed bridges. (*L*) Occlusal view of the maxillary ridge reconstructed with fixed bridges. (*M, N*) Postoperative periapical radiographs of the dental implants and reconstructed maxillary ridge.

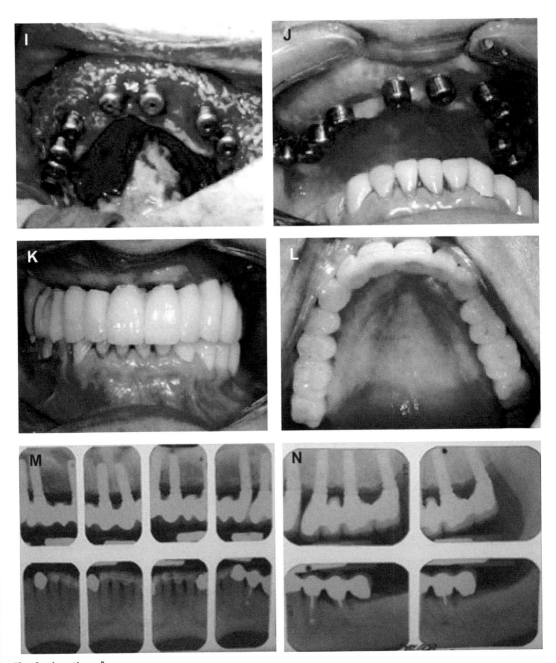

Fig. 6. (*continued*)

hemi trays to protect the graft in this location. The mesh is filled with the chosen bone graft material and secured into position with at least 2 screws on the facial surface of each hemi tray and 1 screw on the lingual, usually in the anterior region just above the genial tubercles. If an additional midline piece of mesh is needed to cover the graft, it can be secured on the facial surface and on the lingual surface with screws. The closure of the incision is performed in 2 layers as previously described.

An extraoral approach can also be used when augmenting the mandible (**Fig. 9**). This incision is made under sterile conditions along the submental crease. The incision must be extended along the full length of the submental crease to achieve adequate exposure. This dissection is carried sharply down to the inferior border of the mandible where a subperiosteal dissection is performed to expose the facial and superior aspect of the mandible. Using this approach the mental nerves

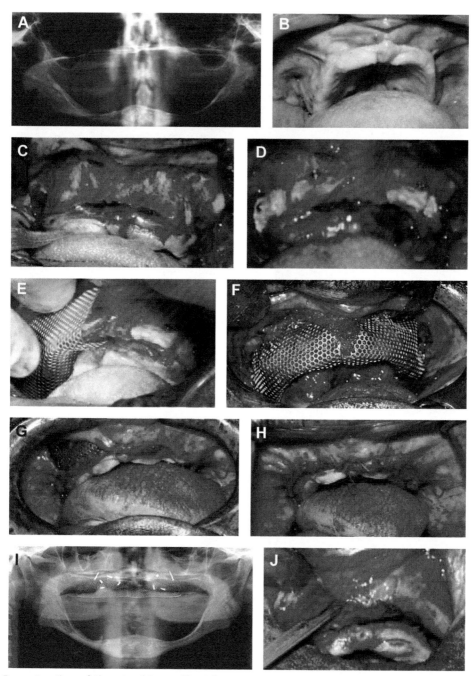

Fig. 7. Reconstruction of the atrophic maxilla. (*A*) Preoperative panoramic radiograph showing an atrophic maxilla. (*B*) Preoperative intraoral view of atrophic maxilla. Exposure of the maxilla through a vestibular incision. (*C*) Note bilateral sinus lifts have been performed. (*D*) Placement of autogenous block grafts onto the anterior maxilla. (*E*) Contouring of the titanium mesh. (*F*) Titanium mesh and bone graft in place secured with screws. (*G, H*) Closure of the maxillary vestibular incision with a horizontal mattress Vicryl suture. (*I*) Postoperative panoramic radiograph with titanium mesh in place. (*J, K*) Exposure of the titanium mesh through a crestal incision. (*L*) Reconstructed maxillary ridge with pseudoperiosteum in place. (*M*) Dental implants placed in the reconstructed maxilla. (*N*) Panoramic radiograph showing dental implants in place. (*O*) Exposure of dental implants and harvest of palatal graphs. (*P*) Vestibuloplasty and placement of palatal graphs. (*Q*) Reconstructed maxillary ridge after gingival grafts have healed. (*R*) Implant-supported fixed-detachable prosthesis in place.

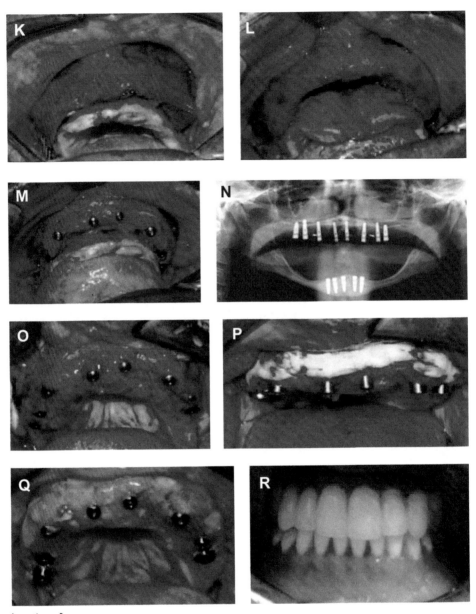

Fig. 7. (*continued*)

can be easily identified. When there is a dehiscence of the inferior alveolar nerve, the neurovascular bundle can be mobilized and transposed posteriorly. In cases where there is no dehiscence, the inferior alveolar nerve transpositioning must be performed to achieve adequate mobilization of the mental nerve and provide adequate room for the titanium mesh trays.[20,23] Once the inferior alveolar nerve is transposed, usually to the second molar region, the titanium mesh tray can be contoured and trimmed. The posterior extent of the inferior aspect of the tray is just anterior to the exit of the inferior alveolar neurovascular bundle. The superior aspect of the tray can extend posteriorly to the retromolar region. The mucosa must be fully mobilized in the retromolar pad region and on the lingual aspect of the mandible to prevent pinching or tearing of the mucosa. Once the mesh has been properly contoured and fitted, it can be filled with the desired bone graft material. It is secured back into position with at least 2 screws in each hemi tray on the facial surface of the mandible and 1 screw on the lingual aspect just above the genial tubercle. The soft tissue is re-draped into position. The vestibule can be secured and deepened at this time using a suturing technique

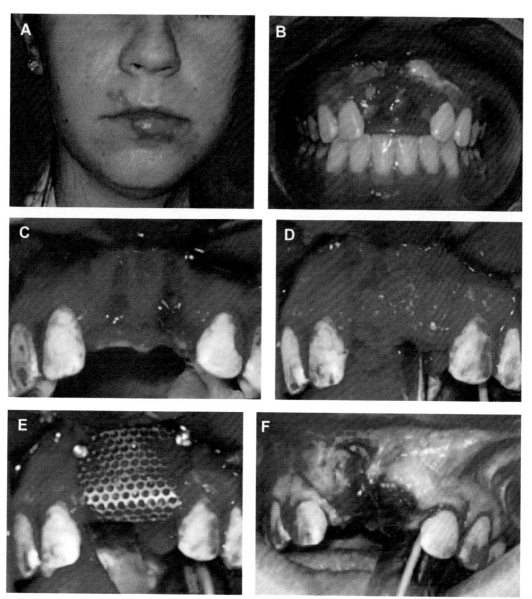

Fig. 8. Segmental defect in the anterior maxilla reconstructed with titanium mesh. (*A, B*) Preoperative views of a patient after trauma resulted in avulsion of maxillary central incisors. (*C*) Exposure of the anterior maxilla through a crestal incision. Note the loss of anterior maxillary alveolar bone. (*D*) Autogenous bone graft in place. (*E*) Titanium mesh in place to protect the bone graft. (*F*) Closure of the grafted site. (*G*) Temporization of the area of 8 and 9. (*H*) Anterior maxillary ridge before mesh removal. (*I*) Surgical exposure of the anterior maxilla to remove the mesh. (*J*) Reconstructed anterior maxilla after mesh removal. (*K*) Implant placement in areas 8 and 9.

described by Bosker and Wardle.[36] Vestibular recreation or re-draping is performed using a 2.0 Vicryl suture placed in a submucosal fashion at the desired depth of the vestibule superiorly. This is sutured inferiorly to the periosteum and musculature along the inferior lingual aspect of the mandible. The second layer is placed at the level of the mentalis muscle superiorly and secured to the digastric musculature inferiorly. The platysma muscle is then closed. In most patients some of the overlying skin along the incision can be excised in a lazy W-fashion to improve the contour of the neck (**Fig. 10**).[36]

Partially Edentulous Mandible

The reconstruction of the partially edentulous mandible is similar to the technique described

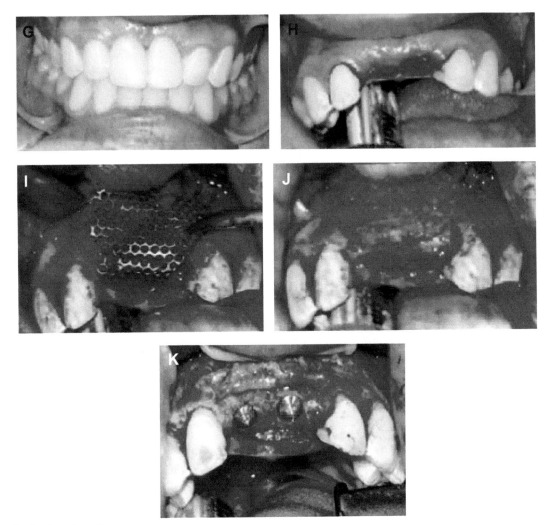

Fig. 8. (continued)

for the partially edentulous maxilla. A vestibular incision is used for exposure, extending toward the line angle on either side of the edentulous space. The incision is extended to near the junction of the attached mucosa. Mobilization of the facial, crestal, and lingual aspect of the soft tissues is usually performed. The dissection around the cervical portion of the teeth is performed in a tunneling fashion subperiosteally to mobilize the gingival cuff. As an alternative to a vestibular incision, a crestal incision can be used in conjunction with a releasing incision at least 2 teeth on either side of the defect. Once the ridge is exposed, the titanium mesh can be trimmed and contoured to fit into position. It is then filled with the desired bone graft material, placed into position, and secured with at least 2 screws on the facial aspect. When a crestal incision is used for exposure, the periosteum must

be released along the facial vestibule to facilitate a tension-free closure of the wound. This is usually not necessary when a vestibular incision is used. Closure is performed in layers with 3.0 Vicryl suture material placed deep to the mucosa. The mucosa is closed with 4.0 Vicryl or Monocryl suture (see **Fig. 9**).

POSTOPERATIVE CARE

The postoperative care includes use of antibiotics such as amoxicillin or clindamycin for 7 to 10 days. Patients are asked to use a chlorhexadine mouth rinse for at least the first 2 to 4 weeks. If wound dehiscence develops, the patient is maintained on chlorhexadine mouth rinse until the time of mesh removal. Appropriate cleaning of the titanium mesh, if exposed, should also include use of a soft toothbrush to remove any plaque or

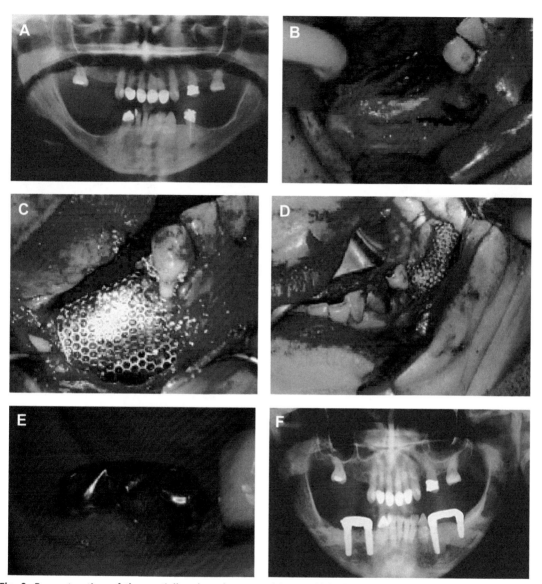

Fig. 9. Reconstruction of the partially edentulous atrophic mandible. (*A*) Preoperative radiograph of partially edentulous atrophic mandible. (*B*) Exposure of the posterior mandible with nerve repositioning. (*C*) Titanium mesh and bone graft in place on the right side of the mandible. (*D*) Titanium mesh and bone graft in place on the left side of the mandible. (*E*) Final restoration in place. (*F*) Postoperative radiograph after reconstruction of the posterior edentulous mandible with titanium mesh, bone grafts, nerve repositioning, and dental implants.

debris. Irrigating the exposed area is desirable. Follow-up visits are usually at 2 weeks, 1 month, 3 months, and 6 months postoperatively.

MESH REMOVAL AND IMPLANT PLACEMENT

The patient is allowed to heal for a period of 4 to 6 months before mesh removal and implant placement. At the time of removal of the mesh, 1 of 2 techniques can be used. The mesh is typically removed from an intraoral approach using a crestal incision. The mesh is easily exposed in a subperiosteal fashion using a sharp periosteal elevator to detach the overlying mucosa. Once it is fully exposed, the mesh can be removed. The screws are removed first, then a periosteal elevator is placed underneath the mesh with the blade of the instrument turned toward the mesh. This facilitates removal and detaching the pseudoperiosteum from the mesh (see **Fig. 6**). The implants are placed using a surgical guide, because it allows for minimal dissection of the soft tissue overlying the ridge. In this technique, if minimal elevation of the pseudoperiosteum is

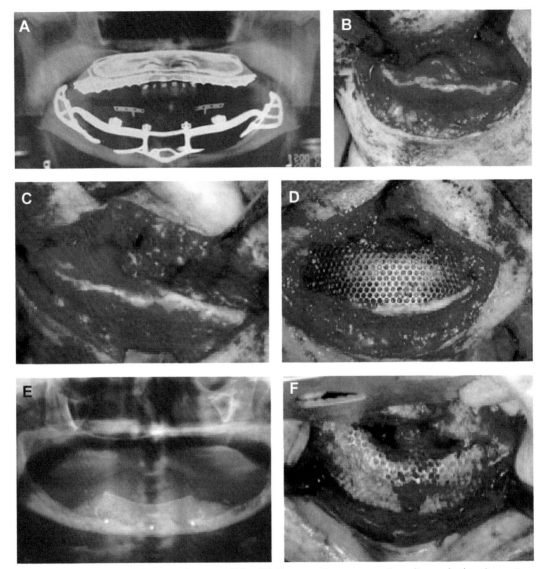

Fig. 10. Reconstruction of the atrophic mandible. (*A*) Preoperative panoramic radiograph showing extreme mandibular atrophy and a failing subperiosteal implant. (*B, C*) Exposure of the mandible through a submental incision. (*D*) Mesh and bone graft in place. (*E*) Postoperative panoramic radiograph showing the mesh and bone graft in place. (*F*) Exposure of the mesh and bone graft through an intraoral approach. (*G*) Grafted mandible with mesh removed. (*H*) Grafted mandible with implants in place. (*I*) Immediate postoperative panoramic radiograph with implants in place. (*J*) Intraoral view after implants have been exposed and palatal graft has been placed. (*K*) Implants have been restored with a bar superstructure. (*L*) Postoperative panoramic radiograph after implants have been restored.

performed, limiting the dissection to the crest of the ridge, a simultaneous vestibuloplasty can be performed at this time. This is done leaving the pseudoperiosteum exposed and suturing the soft tissue that was at the crest of the ridge down to the depth of the vestibule. If this is the planned technique in the maxilla, the initial incision can be made palatal to the crest of the ridge allowing for approximately 4 to 5 mm of the keratinized palatal tissue to be transposed onto the facial surface and

secured in this position. This procedure allows keratinized tissue to be placed along the facial surface and thins the thickened palatal tissue for future ease of cleaning of the dental implants.

The second technique that can be used once the mesh is removed is to elevate the pseudoperiosteum via a crestal incision. This procedure allows for inspection of the newly augmented bone. This dissection should be kept to a minimum to decrease the risk of resorption of the grafted

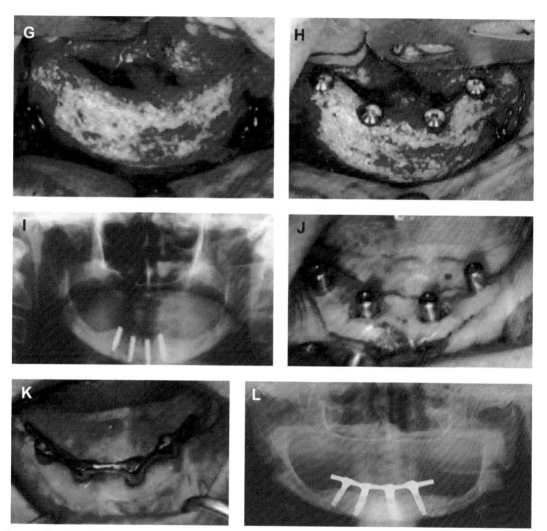

Fig. 10. (*continued*)

bone. When this technique is used, some of the bone may be exposed as a result of tearing of the pseudoperiosteum that may occur during elevation. It is also usually difficult to re-approximate this tissue into the desired position. Primary closure of the wound is performed by re-approximating the elevated mucosa along the crest of the ridge. A vestibuloplasty will need to be performed at the time of implant uncovery. The vestibuloplasty can be performed in a similar fashion as described earlier, leaving the exposed periosteum to heal by secondary intention. A preferred technique is to transfer the thickened palatal mucosa onto the facial surface during the vestibuloplasty, either as a free graft or as a flap.

EXPERIENCE WITH TITANIUM MESH

In 2008, Louis and colleagues[20] reported the use of titanium mesh for vertical ridge augmentation in 44 patients. Of the 44 patients treated, the mean augmentation height was 13.7 mm. The mean healing time between placement of the bone graft and removal of the mesh was 6.9 months. A total of 174 implants were placed in 36 of the 44 patients. This was equally distributed between the maxilla and mandible. The success of the bone graft procedure was 97.72%; 1 patient had complete bone loss. Seven patients declined to have implant placement for financial reasons. Three implants were removed in 1 patient during a mean follow-up time of 17.2 months. A consistent finding during the healing phase was a tendency for dehiscence of the wound and exposure of the mesh. The rate of dehiscence was 52.27% in the 44 patients treated. Seven of these exposures required early removal of the mesh because of infection. In 1 of these patients, complete bone loss occurred as a result of infection.

DISCUSSION

When managing the edentulous maxilla, the clinician is often faced with a large pneumitized maxillary sinus and a very thin alveolar ridge in the anterior maxilla. Alveolar bone resorption can be accelerated with denture use, resulting in loss of vertical height and very thin bone separating the crest of the ridge from the large sinus and the floor of the nose.[2] These patients could be treated in a conventional fashion with augmentation of the sinuses only. When this is done, the patient can be restored with implant-supported dentures or a fixed-detachable prosthesis but the lost vertical dimension must be replaced with acrylic. To improve the implant-to-tooth ratio, vertical augmentation is desired. If near ideal ridge height is obtained, the dentist and patient have several restorative options.

The severely atrophic mandible is also challenging to restore. Placement of implants in the severely atrophic mandible can result in fracture, thus reconstruction with bone grafting is usually indicated. With larger bone stock, implants can sometimes be placed posterior to the mental foramina, allowing for restorative options other than placement of implants in the anterior mandible only.

The use of titanium mesh as a barrier with particulate bone graft has several advantages.[20] The material is nonresorbable and rigid. The rigidity allows for shape maintenance, which is important when attempting to extend the bony envelope. The soft tissue is placed under tension during an augmentation procedure, thus causing a flattening or deforming of nonrigid membranes and the associated graft. Titanium mesh is rigid and will maintain its shape. It is also nonresorbable and will remain present throughout the healing phase of the bone graft. This is important in preventing resorption of the graft during the healing phase.[33,35]

The material is biocompatible and can be placed subperiosteally as a barrier with little or no soft-tissue reaction. Because the mesh has a tendency to become exposed during the healing phase, it is important that the material does not exacerbate or increase this tendency.

The main disadvantages of this material are the cost and the tendency to become exposed during the healing phase. Although the risk of exposure is high, the risk of infection remains low.[20,27] With local wound management, exposure can be tolerated long enough for the graft to mature. The use of a vestibular incision has been used in some cases in an attempt to reduce the risk of dehiscence of the wound. It is unclear at this time if the vestibular incision reduces the risk of wound dehiscence. When a large augmentation is planned, the vestibular approach also allows the incision, when closed, to be at or just to the facial aspect of the crest of the ridge.

Another disadvantage of this technique is the large volume of autogenous bone required to augment an entire ridge. Experience with autogenous bone and resorbable hydroxyapatite or tricalcium phosphate has been positive but it requires harvesting from a distant site such as the tibia or the ileum, with its associated donor site morbidity.

Recent reports using Infuse (Medtronic, Minneapolis, MN) and mineralized and demineralized bone matrix have shown promise.[37–39] Currently, it is unclear whether this material is suitable for replacement of autogenous bone using this technique. Potential advantages of using Infuse may be the avoidance of harvesting autogenous bone and the possibility of enhanced soft-tissue healing with a reduced risk of membrane exposure.

SUMMARY

The use of titanium mesh and autogenous bone graft has been a successful technique for reconstruction of the atrophic maxilla and mandible. The technique can be used in the edentulous and partially edentulous ridge. The main advantage is the rigidity of the material, which prevents collapse and flattening of the graft during vertical ridge augmentation. The material is also nonresorbable and remains present throughout the healing phase of the bone graft.

REFERENCES

1. US Department of Health and Human Services. Oral health in America: a report of the surgeon general. Rockville (MD): US Department of Health and Human Services, National Institutes of Health, National Institute of Dental and Craniofacial Research; 2000.
2. Friedman S. Comparative analysis of the conflicting factors in the selection of occlusal patterns for edentulous patients. J Prosthet Dent 1964;14:30–6.
3. Rodd HD, Malhotra R, O'Brien CH, et al. Change in supporting tissue following loss of a permanent maxillary incisor in children. Dent Traumatol 2007; 23(6):328–32.
4. Louis P, Holmes J, Fernandes R. Resorbable mesh as a containment system in reconstruction of the atrophic mandible fracture. J Oral Maxillofac Surg 2004;62(6):719–23.
5. Bedrossian E, Stumpel L III, Beckely ML, et al. The zygomatic implant: preliminary data on treatment

of severely resorbed maxillae. A clinical report. Int J Oral Maxillofac Implants 2002;17(6):861–5.

6. Deporter D, Watson P, Pharoah M, et al. Five- to 6-year results of a prospective clinical trial using the ENDOPORE dental implant and a mandibular overdenture. Clin Oral Implants Res 1999;10(2):95–102.

7. Diaz-Romeral-Bautista M, Manchon-Miralles A, Asenjo-Cabezon J, et al. Autogenous calvarium bone grafting as a treatment for severe bone resorption in the upper maxilla: a case report. Med Oral Patol Oral Cir Bucal 2009;15(2):e361–65.

8. Griffin TJ, Cheung WS. The use of short, wide implants in posterior areas with reduced bone height: a retrospective investigation. J Prosthet Dent 2004;92(2):139–44.

9. Gutta R, Waite PD. Outcomes of calvarial bone grafting for alveolar ridge reconstruction. Int J Oral Maxillofac Implants 2009;24(1):131–6.

10. Gutta R, Waite PD. Cranial bone grafting and simultaneous implants: a submental technique to reconstruct the atrophic mandible. Br J Oral Maxillofac Surg 2008;46(6):477–9.

11. Hallman M, Nordin T. Sinus floor augmentation with bovine hydroxyapatite mixed with fibrin glue and later placement of nonsubmerged implants: a retrospective study in 50 patients. Int J Oral Maxillofac Implants 2004;19(2):222–7.

12. Hwang SJ, Jung JG, Jung JU, et al. Vertical alveolar bone distraction at molar region using lag screw principle. J Oral Maxillofac Surg 2004;62(7):787–94.

13. Jensen J, Simonsen EK, Sindet-Pedersen S. Reconstruction of the severely resorbed maxilla with bone grafting and osseointegrated implants: a preliminary report. J Oral Maxillofac Surg 1990;48(1):27–32 [discussion: 33].

14. Jensen OT. Alveolar segmental "sandwich" osteotomies for posterior edentulous mandibular sites for dental implants. J Oral Maxillofac Surg 2006;64(3): 471–5.

15. Jensen OT, Block M. Alveolar modification by distraction osteogenesis. Atlas Oral Maxillofac Surg Clin North Am 2008;16(2):185–214.

16. Jensen OT, Ellis E. The book flap: a technical note. J Oral Maxillofac Surg 2008;66(5):1010–4.

17. Jensen OT, Kuhlke L, Bedard JF, et al. Alveolar segmental sandwich osteotomy for anterior maxillary vertical augmentation prior to implant placement. J Oral Maxillofac Surg 2006;64(2):290–6.

18. Laster Z, Rachmiel A, Jensen OT. Alveolar width distraction osteogenesis for early implant placement. J Oral Maxillofac Surg 2005;63(12):1724–30.

19. Lorenzoni M, Pertl C, Polansky R, et al. Guided bone regeneration with barrier membranes–a clinical and radiographic follow-up study after 24 months. Clin Oral Implants Res 1999;10(1):16–23.

20. Louis PJ, Gutta R, Said-Al-Naief N, et al. Reconstruction of the maxilla and mandible with particulate bone graft and titanium mesh for implant placement. J Oral Maxillofac Surg 2008;66(2):235–45.

21. Schmidt BL, Pogrel MA, Young CW, et al. Reconstruction of extensive maxillary defects using zygomaticus implants. J Oral Maxillofac Surg 2004;62(9 Suppl 2):82–9.

22. Waite PD, Sastravaha P, Lemons JE. Biologic mechanical advantages of 3 different cranial bone grafting techniques for implant reconstruction of the atrophic maxilla. J Oral Maxillofac Surg 2005; 63(1):63–7.

23. Louis PJ. Inferior alveolar nerve repositioning. Atlas Oral Maxillofac Surg Clin North Am 2001; 9(2):93–128.

24. Gargiulo EA, Ziter WD, Messina JR, et al. Use of titanium mesh and autogenous bone marrow in the repair of a nonunited mandibular fracture: report of case and review of the literature. J Oral Surg 1973; 31(5):371–6.

25. Cobetto GA, McClary SA, Zallen RD. Treatment of mandibular fractures with malleable titanium mesh plates: a review of 120 cases. J Oral Maxillofac Surg 1983;41(9):597–600.

26. Boyne PJ, Cole MD, Stringer D, et al. A technique for osseous restoration of deficient edentulous maxillary ridges. J Oral Maxillofac Surg 1985;43(2):87–91.

27. Eisig SB, Ho V, Kraut R, et al. Alveolar ridge augmentation using titanium micromesh: an experimental study in dogs. J Oral Maxillofac Surg 2003; 61(3):347–53.

28. Gongloff RK, Cole M, Whitlow W, et al. Titanium mesh and particulate cancellous bone and marrow grafts to augment the maxillary alveolar ridge. Int J Oral Maxillofac Surg 1986;15(3):263–8.

29. von Arx T, Hardt N, Wallkamm B. The TIME technique: a new method for localized alveolar ridge augmentation prior to placement of dental implants. Int J Oral Maxillofac Implants 1996; 11(3):387–94.

30. von Arx T, Kurt B. Implant placement and simultaneous peri-implant bone grafting using a micro titanium mesh for graft stabilization. Int J Periodontics Restorative Dent 1998;18(2):117–27.

31. Baker RD, Terry BC, Davis WH, et al. Long-term results of alveolar ridge augmentation. J Oral Surg 1979;37(7):486–9.

32. Dahlin C, Sandberg E, Alberius P, et al. Restoration of mandibular nonunion bone defects. An experimental study in rats using an osteopromotive membrane method. Int J Oral Maxillofac Surg 1994;23(4):237–42.

33. Rasmusson L, Meredith N, Sennerby L. Measurements of stability changes of titanium implants with exposed threads subjected to barrier membrane induced bone augmentation. An experimental study in the rabbit tibia. Clin Oral Implants Res 1997;8(4): 316–22.

34. Simion M, Trisi P, Piattelli A. Vertical ridge augmentation using a membrane technique associated with osseointegrated implants. Int J Periodontics Restorative Dent 1994;14(6):496–511.

35. Rasmusson L, Meredith N, Kahnberg KE, et al. Effects of barrier membranes on bone resorption and implant stability in onlay bone grafts. An experimental study. Clin Oral Implants Res 1999;10(4):267–77.

36. Bosker H, Wardle ML. Muscular reconstruction to improve the deterioration of facial appearance and speech caused by mandibular atrophy: technique and case reports. Br J Oral Maxillofac Surg 1999;37(4):277–84.

37. Toriumi DM, O'Grady K, Horlbeck DM, et al. Mandibular reconstruction using bone morphogenetic protein 2: long-term follow-up in a canine model. Laryngoscope 1999;109(9):1481–9.

38. Smeets R, Maciejewski O, Gerressen M, et al. Impact of rhBMP-2 on regeneration of buccal alveolar defects during the osseointegration of transgingival inserted implants. Oral Surg Oral Med Oral Pathol Oral Radiol Endod 2009;108(4):e3–e12.

39. Whitesides LM, Radwan A, Sharawy M. Sinus floor augmentation using a composite graft of bone morphogenic protein-2 and allogenic cancellous bone (Puros): case report. J Oral Implantol 2006;32(5):259–64.

Alveolar Distraction Osteogenesis for Dental Implant Preparation: An Update

Luis G. Vega, DDS[a],*, Arturo Bilbao, MD, PhD[b,c]

KEYWORDS

- Alveolar distraction • Alveolar reconstruction
- Dental implants • Bone grafting

Current standards in implant dentistry are intended to provide natural prosthetic restorations with the finest esthetic and functional outcomes. Several parameters have been suggested to achieve gold-standard results: adequate bone height, width, and anteroposterior projection; adequate soft tissue quantity and quality; preservation of buccal sulcus; and adequate papillae and gingival contour.[1] The preservation and reconstruction of the alveolar bone and surrounding soft tissues for the placement of dental implants has become fundamental in the contemporary practice of oral and maxillofacial surgery. As described elsewhere in this issue, multiple techniques have been used for these purposes.

Since its introduction in 1996,[2] alveolar distraction osteogenesis has been considered a viable technique for reconstruction of alveolar bone before implant placement. In 2004, the *Oral and Maxillofacial Clinics of North America* published an article on alveolar distraction osteogenesis. Batal and Cottrell[3] comprehensively reviewed the history, biologic principles, devices, clinical applications, and surgical techniques in alveolar distraction osteogenesis, and readers are referred to this text for the basic concepts on alveolar distraction. This article discusses newer research and provides clinical advice on the practice of alveolar distraction osteogenesis.

BIOLOGY OF ALVEOLAR DISTRACTION OSTEOGENESIS

Alveolar distraction osteogenesis uses biologic principles described in the orthopedic literature.[4,5] After performing an alveolar bone osteotomy, a distractor device is placed in the transport segment, which remains fully vascularized via its periosteum. Subsequently, the bony segment is subjected to gradual traction that separates it from the basal bone; this traction activates tissue growth and regeneration, forming a distraction callus that progressively matures into bone. The resultant bone mass and shape depends on the vector of distraction, mechanical forces, and the blood supply.

Several biologic processes occur during and after distraction. In recent years, several publications have reported specifically on the biology of human alveolar distraction osteogenesis.[6–11] Chiapasco and colleagues[8] reported that, after 12 weeks of consolidation, the percentage of mineralized bone that formed in the distracted

[a] Division of Oral & Maxillofacial Surgery, Department of Surgery, Health Science Center at Jacksonville, University of Florida, 653-1 West 8th Street, Jacksonville, FL 32209, USA
[b] Santiago de Compostela University Hospital, Travesía da Choupana s/n, 15706 Santiago de Compostela, La Coruña, Spain
[c] Private Practice, La Rosaleda Hospital Policlínico, Santiago León de Caracas, 1, 15701 Santiago de Compostela, La Coruña, Spain
* Corresponding author.
E-mail address: luis.vega@jax.ufl.edu

Oral Maxillofacial Surg Clin N Am 22 (2010) 369–385
doi:10.1016/j.coms.2010.04.004
1042-3699/10/$ – see front matter © 2010 Elsevier Inc. All rights reserved.

region ranged from 21.6% to 57.8%. The newly formed bone was oriented perpendicular to the osteotomy cut and consisted of woven bone reinforced by parallel-fibered bone. Türker and colleagues[10] reported similar histologic findings after 12 weeks of consolidation. They also correlated those findings with panoramic radiographs, dental computed tomography (CT) scans, and bone density analysis. Panoramic radiographs at the end of distraction showed radiolucent gaps; after 12 weeks the distraction gaps appeared to be mostly radio-opaque with some radiolucent areas, and after 1 year the appearances were the same as the preexisting bone. Dental CT scans taken 12 weeks after distraction confirmed the increase of alveolar heights and filling of the distraction chamber; after 1 year the CT scans showed formation of bone that appeared similar to preexisting bone. Bone density analysis from the dental CT showed that the newly formed bone after 12 weeks of consolidation was denser than medullary bone. Iizuka and colleagues[6] found that a bidirectional alveolar distractor formed high-density new bone with complex architecture. The new bone was oriented in several different layers. They concluded that the favorable bone regeneration was achieved as a result of the combination of slow distraction and gradual anterior angulation.

Consolo and colleagues[7] compared the use of traditional alveolar distraction with an intermittent loading alveolar distraction. After reaching the distraction goal, the individual started an activation-deactivation protocol for 8 weeks during the consolidation phase. The histologic results at 6, 8, and 12 weeks of consolidation showed evidence of early bone formation with superior structure quality.

Adequate blood supply is crucial for the development, remodeling, and regeneration of bone. Amir and colleagues[9] found a positive correlation between blood vessel volume and bone volume density in newly formed bone after alveolar distraction. This finding supports the concept that vascularity is necessary for the formation of new bone.

Lindeboom and colleagues[11] reported on the vascular density changes in oral mucosa after alveolar distraction. They showed that the main increase of vascularity was during the activation phase. The vessel density during consolidation was comparable with preoperative levels.

DISTRACTION PROTOCOL

After almost 15 years of widespread use, there is still controversy regarding the best protocol. As new devices and applications have been designed, different distraction protocols have been tested and established. However, the original clinical phases of distraction remain the same: osteotomy, latency, distraction, and consolidation (**Fig. 1**).

Osteotomy

Osteotomy has traditionally been performed with rotary burs, different kinds of saws, and osteotomes. Piezosurgery for alveolar distraction osteotomies has also been reported in the literature.[12,13] By comparing piezoelectric with conventional osteotomies for alveolar distraction, González-García and colleagues[13] found that the surgical difficulty and the incidence of intraoperative complications were significantly lower in the piezoelectric group. Their results showed that the postdistraction alveolar morphology was worse in the piezoelectric group. They theorize that the piezoelectric osteotomies will create a wider initial gap that may favor the appearance of granulation tissue without good osteogenic potential.

Latency Period

Latency period is defined as time from surgery to the beginning of distraction. In an alveolar distraction systematic review from 1996 to 2006, the most common latency period was 7 days (66% of the cases reviewed) to allow for healing of the mucoperiosteum and reduce the risk of wound

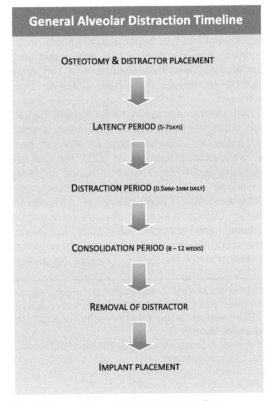

Fig. 1. General alveolar distraction timeline.

dehiscence. Extended latency periods of more than 15 days were applied to ensure complete revascularization of the transport segment in cases in which the mucoperiosteal pedicle is small or endangered.[14]

Distraction Period

The distraction period encompasses the time between initial activation and end of the activation of the distractor device. The amount of distraction required is generally based on the amount of tissue necessary to fulfill the implant and dental rehabilitation goals. Several studies have focused on the amount of alveolar distraction relapse, and their recommendation is to overcorrect by 20% to 25%.[15,16] Apart from the amount of distraction needed, the distraction rate and rhythm are of paramount importance during this period.

Distraction rate

The daily amount of bone to be distracted is known as distraction rate. Saulacic and colleagues[14] reported in a systematic review that the mean distraction rate was 0.71 ($\pm$0.27) mm. They also noted a lower distraction rate of 0.4 to 0.5 mm in cases in which distractor implants and horizontal distraction were used. According to Amir and colleagues,[17] a distraction rate of 0.5 mm per day results in faster osteogenesis than a distraction rate of 1 mm in elderly patients.

Distraction rhythm

Distraction rhythm is the number of distraction activations per day. According to Saulacic and colleagues,[14] the rhythm in alveolar distraction has tended to be chosen empirically, in part because of a lack of experimental findings. They reviewed 209 distractions in 197 patients, and found that the rhythm of distraction ranged between 1 (62%), 2 (35%), and 4 times daily (3%).

Consolidation Period

This is the period that allows for maturation and corticalization of the regenerated bone. According to Amir and colleagues,[9] a minimum of 10 weeks is required for new bone to bridge a 10 mm alveolar distraction gap. It has been suggested that the poorly mineralized bone tissue found after 10 weeks of consolidation will start an adaptive response that would increase the bone matrix mineralization with placement of dental implants.[18] A systematic review found that the mean consolidation period was 12.22 ($\pm$5.58) weeks. A difference was noted in the consolidation period when different distractor devices were used. The mean consolidation period on intraosseous distractors was 8.82 ($\pm$2.67) weeks, 11.44 ($\pm$2.55) weeks for the extraosseous distractors, and 18.02 ($\pm$3.50) weeks before prosthetic treatment started in distraction implants.

ALVEOLAR DISTRACTION DEVICES

Novel alveolar distraction designs are constantly being developed for research and clinical purposes. As a general rule they have been classified as intraosseous and extraosseous, depending on the placement in relation to the bone. In a study comparing clinical outcomes of intraosseous and extraosseous alveolar distractors, Uckan and colleagues,[19] found no significant statistical difference despite the higher complication rate and lower implant success in the intraosseous group. Devices can also be categorized as unidirectional and multidirectional, depending on the direction of the movement. Initial alveolar distractor designs allowed for only a unidirectional movement, making correct positioning of the device and vector control most important. Recent publications have shown the clinical value of multi directional alveolar distraction devices.[6,20,21] A retrospective study comparing outcomes of unidirectional and bidirectional distractor devices, Schleier and colleagues[21] found no significant statistical differences in the bone gain or implant success. Moreover, several cases with unidirectional distraction had to be bone grafted at the time of implant placement. They concluded that this difference was caused by the precise control of the distraction process in the bidirectional distraction group.

INDICATIONS FOR ALVEOLAR DISTRACTION OSTEOGENESIS

Several clinical indications for alveolar distraction osteogenesis have been reported in the literature (**Box 1**).[22–24] Alveolar reconstruction in preparation for dental implant placement continues to be the

---

Box 1
General applications for alveolar distraction osteogenesis

- Moderate to severe vertical alveolar bone defects
- Segmental deficiencies of the alveolar ridge
- Narrow alveolar ridges
- Adjuvant to other bone graft techniques
- Gradual vertical movement of ankylosed teeth
- Gradual vertical movement of an osseointegrated implant together with the surrounding alveolar bone

most common indication (**Fig. 2**). Reconstruction efforts have used alveolar distraction as a definitive procedure to establish the ideal alveolar ridge or as an adjunctive procedure used to gain bone as part of a larger reconstruction plan. Overall, alveolar distraction offers several advantages compared with other augmentation techniques (**Boxes 2** and **3**).[25]

Alveolar distraction has traditionally been used for vertical augmentation of the alveolar ridge, but horizontal[26–28] and segmental alveolar distraction[29,30] have also been described. The main indication for alveolar distraction is to manage the vertical defects in the anterior maxilla and mandible. Posterior maxillary defects are best addressed with traditional techniques such as sinus lift or bone grafts. Vertical defects of the posterior mandible can be treated with alveolar distraction but, if the defect also has a horizontal component, a more traditional approach with an onlay bone graft or guided tissue regeneration is recommended.[31,32]

To facilitate the evaluation and treatment of vertical alveolar defects, Jensen and Block[33] proposed a classification system in which they defined a class I defect as a mild alveolar vertical

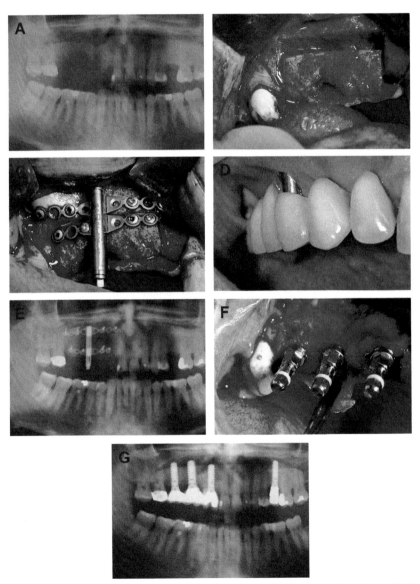

Fig. 2. Alveolar reconstruction using alveolar distraction in preparation for dental implants. (*A*) Right maxillary posttraumatic vertical defect. (*B*) Osteotomy. (*C*) Alveolar distractor in place. (*D*) Vector control using a prosthesis. (*E*) Panoramic radiograph after the end of the distraction. (*F*) Placement of dental implants. (*G*) Panoramic radiograph at the end of the treatment.

Box 2
Advantages of alveolar distraction osteogenesis for preparation for implant placement

- Simple technique
- Simultaneous augmentation of bone and soft tissues
- Less resorption than traditional bone grafts
- Transport segment can include teeth or implants, facilitating the correction of occlusal or prosthetic defects
- Elimination of donor-site morbidity
- Shorter treatment times compared with traditional bone grafting techniques
- Allows the implementation of complementary techniques when results are not optimal

---

deficiency with up to 5 mm that ideally can be treated by a sandwich osteotomy or more traditional bone graft techniques, although distraction can be considered when there are prosthetic concerns in the esthetic zone. Class II defects consist of a moderate vertical loss of 6 to 10 mm that ideally will benefit from alveolar distraction. Class III defects are severe vertical losses greater than 10 mm. Treatment of these defects depends on the available bone stock. If sufficient bone exists, distraction can be carried out first, and definitive alveolar bone form and position can be performed with a bone graft. If the amount of bone is not sufficient for distraction, bone augmentation is carried out first followed by distraction. Vertical defects that involve adjacent teeth with significant bone loss are designated as class IV. In these cases, by extracting the affected dentition, the defect will be converted into a class II or III defect, making the problem more predictable and easier to resolve.

PLANNING FOR ALVEOLAR DISTRACTION OSTEOGENESIS

Clinical examination will establish a preliminary idea of the patient prosthetic needs, occlusion,

---

Box 3
Disadvantages of alveolar distraction osteogenesis for preparation for implant placement

- Patient acceptance and compliance
- Requires careful vector control
- Interference with occlusion might require the construction of protective appliances
- High device cost

---

and the size and shape of the alveolar defect. Maxillary and mandibular models with a diagnostic wax-up will allow corroboration of the clinical findings. They can also be used to fabricate a surgical splint that could be use for vector control as well as temporary restoration. Models also play an important role in planning for the distraction vector, allowing preadaptation of the device, decreasing surgical time, and identifying possible device interferences with opposing dentition. In more complex cases, sterolithographic models are a good option for treatment planning.

Radiographic examination with plain films or CT scan is useful for alveolar defect assessment but it also allows for planning the length and height of the osteotomy. Of great importance is the amount of bone stock and its relationship with the inferior alveolar nerve, inferior border of the mandible, nasal floor, and maxillary sinus. These factors could limit device placement or the distraction procedure. Added consideration should be given to the prophylactic plating of the mandible in which the remaining basal bone is scarce, to prevent fracture and retention of compromised teeth adjacent to the distractor procedure and to help with vector control. Newer technologies, such as computer-assisted surgical planning, are also being applied to alveolar distraction (**Fig. 3**).[34]

ALVEOLAR DISTRACTION: SURGICAL ADVICE

During the different phases of alveolar distraction, there are a series of considerations that can contribute to a successful outcome. Allocating sufficient time for surgical planning is probably the single most important element in alveolar distraction.

Incision

- Special consideration should be given to the location of the incision, because it will affect the quality of the soft tissue that will be augmented at the end of treatment
- Use sound surgical principles that will guarantee proper blood supply to the mucosa and bone
- Careful and conservative dissection will maintain the vascularity of the transport segment, decreasing excessive resorption and avoiding damage to adjacent structures.

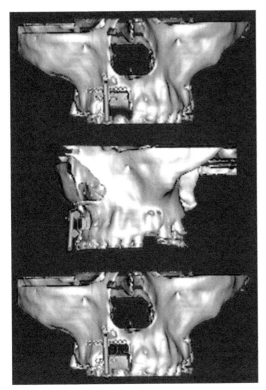

Fig. 3. Alveolar distraction treatment planning using computer-assisted surgical software.

Osteotomy and Distractor Placement

- Use a trapezoidal, semielliptical, or L-shaped osteotomy, depending on location
- Lingually convergent osteotomies will decrease the lingual tipping of the distractor
- A piezoelectric-assisted osteotomy will allow a deeper cut, decreasing the amount of chiseling required
- A transport segment as large as possible (avoiding compromise of basal bone and adjacent structures), and not just containing cortical bone, will avoid a higher rate of resorption
- Newer modular extraosseous distractors will allow the osteotomy to be performed after the placement of the device, because of their ability to remove the distractor rod
- Check that the transport segment is able to move freely through the extension of the distractor (with the exception of L-shaped osteotomy)
- In cases of large transport segments, consider the placement of 2 distraction devices (**Fig. 4**)
- During extraosseous distraction, vector control can be achieved if the distractor

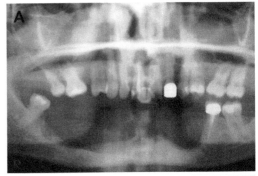

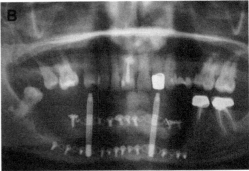

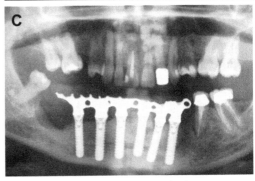

Fig. 4. Placement of 2 distractors for large transport segments. (*A*) Large mandibular defect. (*B*) Placement of 2 distractors. (*C*) Final result after distraction and implant placement.

plate for the transport bone is cut longer than usual, allowing movement along the buccal bone surface.

Distraction Phase

- Decreasing the distraction rate and maintaining good oral hygiene will help in the treatment of wound dehiscence.
- Patients should carry a daily log to record the amount of daily activations.
- Monitor the distraction vector carefully. Several methods for vector control have been described,[35–38] and these are illustrated in **Fig. 5** and **Box 4**.

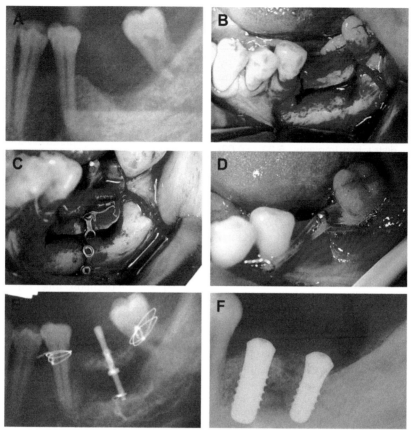

Fig. 5. Vector control. (*A*) Mandibular vertical defect with severe bone loss involving second molar. (*B*) Osteotomy. (*C*) Placement of intraosseous distractor. (*D*, *E*) Vector control using orthodontic elastics and compromised tooth. (*F*) Final result after distraction, extraction of second mandibular molar, and placement of 2 implants.

- When a prosthesis is used as vector control, it must be adjusted daily.
- Always consider overcorrection.

Consolidation Phase

- Covering the distractor rod with a red Robinson catheter will avoid excessive trauma to the surrounding soft tissues

---

Box 4
Methods for vector control in alveolar distraction osteogenesis

- Device modifications
- Orthodontic mechanics: elastic traction, wire stabilization
- Modified prosthesis
- Manual manipulation of the regenerated bone
- Osteotomy after distraction completed

- Avoid excessive pressure on transport segment when using a temporary prosthesis
- In selected cases, implant placement during the consolidation phase will allow for stability of the regenerated bone and maintenance of the distraction vector.

Implant Placement

- Thoroughly clean the granulation tissue in the area where an intraosseous distractor has been placed. Avoid placement of implants in this area but, if necessary, use a large-diameter implant
- When possible, use long implants that will engage the native bone. Implant planning software is helpful in this treatment stage
- To avoid further resorption, do not delay implant loading more than traditional implant protocols.

CLINICAL OUTCOMES IN ALVEOLAR DISTRACTION OSTEOGENESIS
Vertical Bone Gain

Data of 181 patients from a recent review by Chiapasco and colleagues[39] showed that the amount of bone gain after distraction osteogenesis had a range of 3 to 20 mm. Saulacic and colleagues[14] reported in their systematic review the mean bone gain obtained by different types of distractors: distraction implants, 5.02 ($\pm$0.09) mm; intraosseous distractors, 7.86 ($\pm$0.36) mm; and extraosseous distractors, 9.31 ($\pm$0.45) mm. A clinical assessment of 40 patients subjected to an extraosseous distraction showed that the bone augmentation average was 9.5 mm in height, showing a 92.5% success rate.[40] Kanno and colleagues[16] reported comparable results on bone gain using extraosseous distractors; they also noted that, during the consolidation period, there was 15% to 25% bone height reduction. These findings are similar to the previous reports in the literature that recommend 20% to 25% overcorrection in vertical alveolar distraction.[15,41,42] Perdijk and colleagues[43] pointed out the influence of vector of distraction on vertical gain. They studied 34 cases of alveolar distraction on atrophic mandible in which nearly all patients had lingual tipping of the segment by a mean of 12°. This finding meant that, in those cases, only 87% of maximum vertical bone gain could be achieved.

Alveolar Distraction Compared with Conventional Bone Grafting Techniques

In 2004, Chiapasco and colleagues[44] compared alveolar distraction osteogenesis with guided bone regeneration on vertically deficient alveolar ridges. This prospective study evaluated parameters such as bone resorption of the regenerated ridges before and after implant placement, peri-implant bone loss at 1, 2, and 3 years after prosthetic loading of the implant, and success rates of implants. The results suggested that alveolar distraction might offer more predictable long-term results for bone gain maintenance and peri-implant bone resorption. Furthermore, implant success rates were significantly higher in the alveolar distraction group. Chiapasco and colleagues[45] also compared alveolar osteogenesis with autogenous onlay bone grafts using the similar parameters. This study found that bone resorption before implant placement was significantly higher in the autogenous onlay bone graft group. For implant success, no difference was encountered between the groups. Uckan and colleagues[46] also compared alveolar distraction with autogenous onlay graft using complication and implant survival rates. Their results showed a higher complication rate with the alveolar distraction (66.8% vs 33.8%). But they also reported that those complications were minor and easier to treat than those of the autogenous onlay graft. Again, implant survival rates were similar between the groups (91.4% alveolar distraction vs 93.7% autogenous onlay graft). In a prospective study comparing alveolar distraction with inlay bone grafting in the posterior mandible, Bianchi and colleagues[47] showed that, although the mean bone gain with alveolar distraction was significantly better (10 mm vs 5.8 mm), the complication rate was significantly higher in the alveolar distraction group (60%) than in the inlay bone graft group (14.3%).

Two literature reviews of bone augmentation procedures on edentulous ridges for dental implants concluded that it is difficult to demonstrate that one surgical procedure offered better outcomes than another because of the poor methodological quality of the articles published (**Table 1**).[39,48] Their recommendation is to give

Table 1
Comparison of augmentation techniques on edentulous ridges for dental implant placement

Technique	Success Rate (%)	Implant Survival (%)
Guided bone regeneration	60–100	92–100
Onlay bone grafts	92–100	60–100
Split ridge	98–100	91–97.3
Alveolar distraction	96.7–100	90.4–100
Microvascular flaps	87.5	88.2

Data from Chiapasco M, Zaniboni M, Boisco M. Augmentation procedures for the rehabilitation of deficient edentulous ridges with oral implants. Clin Oral Implants Res 2006;17(Suppl 2):136–59.

priority to those procedures that are simpler, less invasive, involve less risk of complications, and reach their goals in the shortest time.

Alveolar Distraction on a Previously Reconstructed Site

Reconstruction of severe maxillary and mandibular defects for dental implants after trauma or tumor ablation is often a difficult task. Case reports in the literature describe the use of alveolar distraction as adjuvant to enhance sites previously reconstructed with iliac bone grafts,[49,50] scapula free flaps,[51,52] and fibular free flaps.[53,54]

In a retrospective study, Kunkel and colleagues[50] reported on 4 patients who underwent iliac crest bone graft for mandibular reconstruction after tumor ablation and later alveolar distraction with an intraosseous device. The vertical gain range was from 5 to 9 mm and, of the 12 implants placed, 1 failed and 1 had critical bone loss after 40 months of follow-up. Hirota and colleagues[51,52] described the use alveolar distraction to enhance the mandibular reconstruction carried out with free scapula flaps in 2 patients. They reported vertical gains of 9 and 10 mm and placement of 9 implants with a 100% success rate after 2 years of follow-up. In 2009, Lizio and colleagues[54] used alveolar distraction to increase the vertical bone height on 6 patients after reconstruction with free fibula flaps. The mean vertical bone gain was 14 mm (12–15 mm). They placed 35 implants, 4 of which failed during the follow-up period, bringing the cumulative implant survival to 89%. They also reported 1 case with fracture of the remaining basal fibula during consolidation.

Success of Dental Implants in Distracted Bone

Prosthetic rehabilitation facilitated by the placement of dental implants is the ultimate goal of alveolar distraction. Controversy still remains regarding the best time for implant placement.

A prospective multicenter study reported the outcomes of 138 implants placed in distracted bone after 2 or 3 months of consolidation. After a mean follow-up of 34 months after prosthetic loading, the success rate was 94.2% with a cumulative survival rate of 100%. No statistically significant differences were found between the different centers.[55]

Using 92 distractor implants on 46 patients with severely atrophic mandibles, Raghoebar and colleagues[56] reported a survival rate of 97% after a minimum of 62 months of follow-up. In a retrospective study, Elo and colleagues[57] compared the implant success rates in distracted bone with autogenous bone-grafted sites. They placed 184 implants on 65 patients reconstructed with autogenous bone, with an implant success rate of 97%. The distraction group contained 56 implants on 17 patients and a success rate of 98%. Again, no statistical difference was noted between groups.

A systematic review on alveolar distraction analyzed a total of 469 implants placed in distracted bone. The mean osseointegration period was 4.59 (±1.34) months. The overall survival rate was 97%. They reported 14 implant failures, 10 of them before loading. The mean follow-up was 14.19 (±11.03) months. This analysis also found no significant difference in implant failure rate associated with location, indication for distraction, latency period, and daily rate and rhythm. The mean augmentation rates approached a statistically significant difference: rate on successful implants was 6.79 (±2.51) mm and 8.40 (±2.31) mm on failed implants. A significant difference was encountered in the relationship between implant failures and distraction implants. Consolidation period also showed significant differences; failed implants were placed after 8.10 (±2.51) weeks, compared with 12.43 (±5.62) weeks for successful implants. Peri-implant bone level was reported for 301 implants. Stable peri-implant bone level was maintained in 285 (95%) of the implants.[14] Recent studies reported peri-implant bone loss values of 0.89 to 1.9 mm/y in areas of alveolar bone distraction.[42,58]

Immediate Loading of Implants on Distracted Bone

In 2004, Degidi and colleagues[59] presented a case of immediate loading of implants placed in distracted bone. Although this practice has not been popular, a study was carried out comparing data from radiofrequency analysis on implants placed in native bone and distracted bone. Even when the results were significantly inferior for implants placed in distracted bone, the investigators concluded that the values obtained suggest the possibility of immediate loading with outcomes similar to those of implants in native bone.[60]

Adjunctive Techniques to Improve the Outcomes of Alveolar Distraction

Research is being conducted on ways to improve the outcome of alveolar distraction. Robiony and colleagues[61] reported on their long-term experience with 12 patients after alveolar distraction and a combination of autologous bone graft with platelet-rich plasma on severely atrophic mandibles. After performing an osteotomy, the distractor

Table 2
Complications of alveolar distraction, possible causes, management and prevention

Phase	Complication	Causes	Management	Prevention
Intraoperative	Inability to mobilize the transport segment	• Incomplete osteotomy • Poor osteotomy design with lack of divergence	Retrace osteotomy	Better execution and planning of the osteotomy
	Fracture of the transport segment	• Lack of sufficient bone stock • Excessive force during mobilization of the osteotomy	Small fractures: removal of fragment, relocate distractor arms to new position (extraosseous devices) (**Fig. 6**) Large fractures: suspension of distraction procedure, osteosynthesis, possible bone graft (**Fig. 7**)	Cautious osteotomy and mobilization of the transport segment
	Fracture of the basal bone	• Lack of sufficient bone stock • Excessive force during mobilization of the osteotomy	Reduction and fixation of fracture segments	Careful planification and execution of osteotomy
	Occlusal interference of distractor rod	• Lack of proper planification	Shortening or reposition of distractor rod	Careful planning using cast models
	Damage to adjacent structures	• Improper surgical technique	Conservative	Careful planning and execution of osteotomy
	Distractor fracture (extraosseous devices)	• Excessive bending of distractor arms	Change distractor device	Use cast models to prebend device avoiding excessive manipulation

Phase	Complication	Causes	Management	Prevention
During distraction and consolidation	Wound dehiscence	• Excessive tension at closure • Poor soft-tissue coverage	Reduction distraction rate, secondary suture	Smaller distraction rate
	Mucosa perforation	• Sharp bony edges in the transport segment	Trimming sharp edge	Smoothing alveolar ridge irregularities
	Premature consolidation	• Lack of compliance of the patient • Excessive latency period • Slow distraction rate	Repeat osteotomy	Correct patient selection and patient education Decrease latency period Increase distraction rate Avoid excessive manipulation of devices
	Distractor failure	• Loosening due to poor bone quality on the transport segment • Distractor fracture	Distractor removal Consider distractor replacement or bone grafting procedure (**Fig. 8**)	
	Incorrect distraction vector	• Excessive pull from lingual and palatal periosteum, muscle insertions • Incorrect placement of the distractor	Vector control (see **Table 1**)	Careful planning, close monitoring
	Transport bone resorption	• Interruption of blood supply due to excessive reflection of perforation of tissue	Consider overcorrection	Conservative
After distraction	Bone defect	• Multifactorial	Consider bone grafting	Good alveolar distraction technique

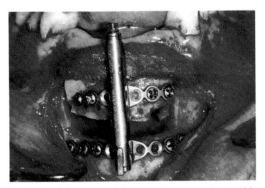

Fig. 6. Small fracture of transport segment treated by repositioning the distractor device.

was activated for 2 to 3 mm and the gap was filled with the combination of iliac crest bone graft and platelet-rich plasma. Their results showed a vertical bone gain that range from 7 to 10 mm with 1 failed case due to scar retraction. The mean decrease of total bone volume was 2.3% at the time of implant placement. A total of 47 implants were placed, and bone loss after 1 year of loading was 0.61 mm and 1.51 mm after 5 years. The implant survival and success rates were 97.9% and 91.5%. A double-blinded trial investigated whether low-intensity pulsed ultrasound therapy stimulates osteogenesis in mandibular

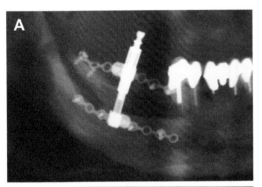

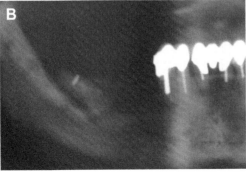

Fig. 7. (*A, B*) Panoramic radiographs showing large fracture of transport segment that required the suspension of the procedure.

alveolar distraction. Biopsies taken at implant placement after 46 ± 8.1 days of consolidation underwent histologic and microradiographic examination. The investigators concluded that ultrasound treatment does not seem to stimulate bone formation.[62] Dergin and colleagues[63] reported a case using a novel technique whereby alveolar distraction was done incorporating a polytetrafloroethylene membrane for protection of the distraction chamber. No defects were noted in the 10 mm of newly regenerated bone. Further research is necessary to validate this technique. At the time of this writing, no human studies using bone morphogenic proteins and alveolar distraction have been published in the English literature.

Patient Perception and Satisfaction After Alveolar Distraction

Even when objective clinical data suggest good results, ultimately it is patient satisfaction that leads to the success of a treatment plan. Using a distractor implant on 46 patients, Raghoebar and colleagues[56] reported patient satisfaction of 8.1 (±1.2) (0 = completely dissatisfied; 10 = completely satisfied) after finalization of the prosthetic treatment. Allais and colleagues[64] used extraosseous devices in 50 patients to evaluate the patients' perceptions during and after alveolar distraction. Their findings showed that, in 76% of the cases, the patient reported the surgery as good and bearable (all patients were orally sedated with 15 mg of midazolam). During distraction, 4% of the patients felt pain, 46% had some difficulty activating the device, and 10% needed extra help. The activation rod was a cause of complaint in 52%. Of the 50 patients, 27 had to undergo additional autologous bone grafting, and 70% of them stated that the bone grafting procedure was more painful than the alveolar distraction. Seventy-eight percent of the patients treated with alveolar distraction would undergo this procedure again if necessary. In a more recent study from the French literature, Castry and colleagues[65] analyzed the answers of 23 patients after alveolar distraction. They found that 87% of the patients adjusted well to the procedure. Light to moderate pain was reported by 57%, and 43% of the patients cataloged the procedure as painful. Fifty-seven percent of the patients managed to forget the presence of the distractor, and 65% had no problem with the length of the treatment. Approximately 91% of the patients were able to activate the distractor device on their own, and 52% of the patients reported that they would undergo another distraction procedure if necessary.

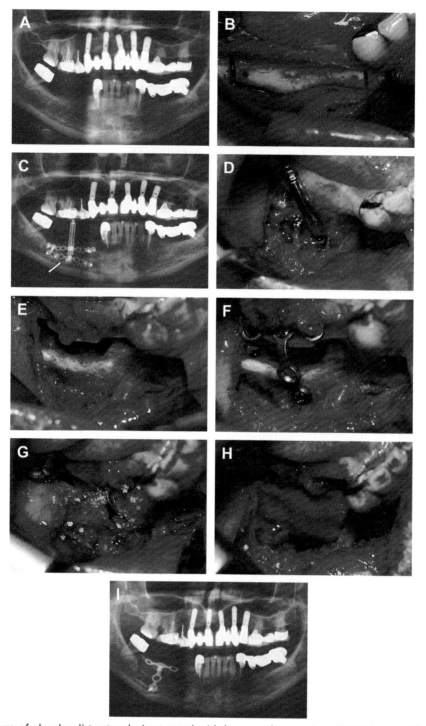

Fig. 8. Fracture of alveolar distractor device treated with bone graft procedure. (*A*) Right mandibular vertical defect. (*B*) Osteotomy. (*C, D*) Panoramic radiograph and clinical picture showing fracture of the alveolar distraction device. (*E*) Distraction gap after removal of device. (*F*) Stabilization of transport segment with miniplates. (*G, H*) Bone graft and membrane in place. (*I*) Radiograph showing vertical bone augmentation.

Complication Rates of Alveolar Distraction

Despite almost 15 years of clinical practice, growing popularity, and newer technologies, alveolar distraction continues to be a challenging procedure. Alveolar distraction complications have conventionally been classified according to the distraction phases in which they occurred: intraoperative, during distraction, during consolidation, and after distraction. They can also be classified as minor complications or major complications that are more difficult to manage and could jeopardize the distraction procedure. In addition to the common complications of any surgical procedure, such as excessive bleeding, hematoma, infection, and paresthesia, there is a set of specific complications for alveolar distraction. These complications, the possible causes, management, and prevention are listed in **Table 2**.

In more recent years, several articles have focus on the complications of alveolar distraction. These studies have reported a wide array of complication rates, ranging from 36% to 100%.[41,42,66–70] In a comprehensive review of the literature from 1996 to 2008, Saulacic and colleagues[71] studied the complication rate of alveolar distraction. Their results showed an overall complication rate of 30%. The most common complication was insufficient bone formation after the consolidation period (8%), followed by regression of distraction distance (7%), and problems related to the device (6%). Intraoperative complications include bleeding from the floor of the mouth (4%) and temporary paresthesia (4%). During the distraction period, wound dehiscence was found on 1% of the patients. Pain was reported in 1% of the patients, as well as mild soft-tissue resistance. Vector deviation was found in 2%. More severe complications were found during the consolidation period, including a mandibular fracture rate of 2% and problems related to the device in 6% of the cases. They also found that insufficient bone formation and evidence of complications were significantly related to the type of distractor and augmentation rates greater than 0.5 mm daily. The investigators concluded that, although complications in alveolar distraction are frequent, they rarely cause severe problems. They suggested that most of the complications could be related to lack of experience and the learning process.

SUMMARY

Alveolar distraction is a technique in constant evolution. A review of the literature within the past 14 years reveal that there are clear indications for its use, with outcomes similar to and sometimes even more predictable than traditional bone grafting techniques in preparation for implant placement. Although complications exist with alveolar distraction, it seems that most are minor and easy to manage. Appropriate patient selection and a better understanding of the technique are paramount in successful bone regeneration with alveolar distraction osteogenesis.

REFERENCES

1. Guerrero C, López P, Figueroa F, et al. Three-dimensional alveolar distraction osteogenesis. In: Bell W, Guerrero C, editors. Distraction osteogenesis of the facial skeleton. 1st edition. Hamilton (Canada): BC Decker; 2007. p. 457–93.
2. Chin M, Toth BA. Distraction osteogenesis in maxillofacial surgery using internal devices: review of five cases. J Oral Maxillofac Surg 1996;54(1):45–53.
3. Batal HS, Cottrell DA. Alveolar distraction osteogenesis for implant site development. Oral Maxillofac Surg Clin North Am 2004;16(1):91–109.
4. Ilizarov GA. The tension-stress effect on the genesis and growth of tissues. Part I. The influence of stability of fixation and soft-tissue preservation. Clin Orthop Relat Res 1989;238:249–81.
5. Ilizarov GA. The tension-stress effect on the genesis and growth of tissues: Part II. The influence of the rate and frequency of distraction. Clin Orthop Relat Res 1989;239:263–85.
6. Iizuka T, Hallermann W, Seto I, et al. Bi-directional distraction osteogenesis of the alveolar bone using an extraosseous device. Clin Oral Implants Res 2005;16(6):700–7.
7. Consolo U, Bertoldi C, Zaffe D. Intermittent loading improves results in mandibular alveolar distraction osteogenesis. Clin Oral Implants Res 2006;17(2):179–87.
8. Chiapasco M, Biglioli F, Autelitano L, et al. Clinical outcome of dental implants placed in fibula-free flaps used for the reconstruction of maxillomandibular defects following ablation for tumors or osteoradionecrosis. Clin Oral Implants Res 2006;17(2):220–8.
9. Amir LR, Becking AG, Jovanovic A, et al. Formation of new bone during vertical distraction osteogenesis of the human mandible is related to the presence of blood vessels. Clin Oral Implants Res 2006;17(4):410–6.
10. Türker N, Basa S, Vural G. Evaluation of osseous regeneration in alveolar distraction osteogenesis with histological and radiological aspects. J Oral Maxillofac Surg 2007;65(4):608–14.
11. Lindeboom JA, Mathura KR, Milstein DMJ, et al. Microvascular soft tissue changes in alveolar distraction osteogenesis. Oral Surg Oral Med Oral Pathol Oral Radiol Endod 2008;106(3):350–5.

12. González-García A, Diniz-Freitas M, Somoza-Martín M, et al. Piezoelectric bone surgery applied in alveolar distraction osteogenesis: a technical note. J Craniofac Surg 2007;22(6):1012–6.

13. González-García A, Diniz-Freitas M, Somoza-Martín M, et al. Piezoelectric and conventional osteotomy in alveolar distraction osteogenesis in a series of 17 patients. Int J Oral Maxillofac Implants 2008;23(5):891–6.

14. Saulacic N, Iizuka T, Martin MS, et al. Alveolar distraction osteogenesis: a systematic review. Int J Oral Maxillofac Surg 2008;37(1):1–7.

15. Saulacic N, Somoza-Martin M, Gándara-Vila P, et al. Relapse in alveolar distraction osteogenesis: an indication for overcorrection. J Oral Maxillofac Surg 2005;63(7):978–81.

16. Kanno T, Mitsugi M, Furuki Y, et al. Overcorrection in vertical alveolar distraction osteogenesis for dental implants. Int J Oral Maxillofac Surg 2007;36(5):398–402.

17. Amir LR, Becking AG, Jovanovic A, et al. Vertical distraction osteogenesis in the human mandible: a prospective morphometric study. Clin Oral Implants Res 2006;17(4):417–25.

18. Marchetti C, Corinaldesi G, Pieri F, et al. Alveolar distraction osteogenesis for bone augmentation of severely atrophic ridges in 10 consecutive cases: a histologic and histomorphometric study. J Periodontol 2007;78(2):360–6.

19. Uckan S, Oguz Y, Bayram B. Comparison of intraosseous and extraosseous alveolar distraction osteogenesis. J Oral Maxillofac Surg 2007;65(4):671–4.

20. Robiony M, Toro C, Stucki-McCormick SU, et al. The "FAD" (Floating Alveolar Device): a bidirectional distraction system for distraction osteogenesis of the alveolar process. J Oral Maxillofac Surg 2004;62(9 Suppl 2):136–42.

21. Schleier P, Wolf C, Siebert H, et al. Treatment options in distraction osteogenesis therapy using a new bidirectional distractor system. J Craniofac Surg 2007;22(3):408–16.

22. Nocini PF, De Santis D, Ferrari F, et al. A customized distraction device for alveolar ridge augmentation and alignment of ankylosed teeth. Int J Oral Maxillofac Implants 2004;19(1):133–44.

23. Mendonça G, Mendonça DB, Fernandes Neto AJ, et al. Use of distraction osteogenesis for repositioning of an osseointegrated implant: a case report. Int J Oral Maxillofac Implants 2008;23(3):551–5.

24. Marcantonio E, Dela Coleta R, Spin-Neto R, et al. Use of a tooth-implant supported bone distractor in oral rehabilitation: description of a personalized technique. J Oral Maxillofac Surg 2008;66(11):2339–44.

25. Bilbao A. Regeneración del proceso alveolar. Rev Esp Cir Oral Maxilofac 2002;24(5):298–303 [in Spanish].

26. Takahashi T, Funaki K, Shintani H, et al. Use of horizontal alveolar distraction osteogenesis for implant placement in a narrow alveolar ridge: a case report. Int J Oral Maxillofac Implants 2004;19(2):291–4.

27. García-García A, Somoza-Martín M, Gandara-Vila P, et al. Horizontal alveolar distraction: a surgical technique with the transport segment pedicled to the mucoperiosteum. J Oral Maxillofac Surg 2004;62(11):1408–12.

28. Gaggl A, Rainer H, Chiari FM. Horizontal distraction of the anterior maxilla in combination with bilateral sinus lift operation – preliminary report. Int J Oral Maxillofac Surg 2005;34(1):37–44.

29. Bilbao A, Cobo R, Hernández M, et al. Reconstrucción del maxilar superior mediante transporte del proceso alveolar. Rev Esp Cir Oral y Maxilofac 2006;28(1):51–6.

30. Basa S, Varol A, Yilmaz S. Transport distraction osteogenesis of a dentoalveolar segment in the posterior mandible: a technical note. J Oral Maxillofac Surg 2007;65(9):1862–4.

31. Louis PJ, Gutta R, Said-Al-Naief N, et al. Reconstruction of the maxilla and mandible with particulate bone graft and titanium mesh for implant placement. J Oral Maxillofac Surg 2008;66(2):235–45.

32. Gutta R, Waite PD. Outcomes of calvarial bone grafting for alveolar ridge reconstruction. Int J Oral Maxillofac Implants 2009;24(1):131–6.

33. Jensen OT, Block M. Alveolar modification by distraction osteogenesis. Atlas Oral Maxillofac Surg Clin North Am 2008;16(2):185–214.

34. Kanno T, Mitsugi M, Sukegawa S, et al. Computer-simulated bi-directional alveolar distraction osteogenesis. Clin Oral Implants Res 2008;19(12):1211–8.

35. Herford AS, Audia F. Maintaining vector control during alveolar distraction osteogenesis: a technical note. Int J Oral Maxillofac Implants 2004;19(5):758–62.

36. García-García A, Peñarrocha-Diago M, Somoza-Martín M, et al. Modified LEAD System distractor to prevent tilting during alveolar distraction in the mandibular symphyseal region. Br J Oral Maxillofac Surg 2008;46(2):141–3.

37. Kilic E, Kilic K, Alkan A. Alternative method to reposition the dislocated transport segment during vertical alveolar distraction. J Oral Maxillofac Surg 2009;67(10):2306–10.

38. Mehra P, Figueroa R. Vector control in alveolar distraction osteogenesis. J Oral Maxillofac Surg 2008;66(4):776–9.

39. Chiapasco M, Casentini P, Zaniboni M. Bone augmentation procedures in implants dentistry. Int J Oral Maxillofac Implants 2009;24(Suppl):237–59.

40. Mazzonetto R, Serra E, Silva FM, et al. Clinical assessment of 40 patients subjected to alveolar distraction osteogenesis. Implant Dent 2005;14(2):149–53.

41. Wolvius EB, Scholtemeijer M, Weijland M, et al. Complications and relapse in alveolar distraction osteogenesis in partially dentulous patients. Int J Oral Maxillofac Surg 2007;36(8):700–5.

42. Ettl T, Gerlach T, Schüsselbauer T, et al. Bone resorption and complications in alveolar distraction osteogenesis. Clin Oral Investig 2009. DOI:10.1007/s00784-009-0340-y.

43. Perdijk FB, Meijer GJ, van Strijen PJ, et al. Effect of extraosseous devices designed for vertical distraction of extreme resorbed mandibles on backward rotation of upper bone segments. Br J Oral Maxillofac Surg 2009;47(1):31–6.

44. Chiapasco M, Romeo E, Casentini P, et al. Alveolar distraction osteogenesis vs. vertical guided bone regeneration for the correction of vertically deficient edentulous ridges: a 1–3-year prospective study on humans. Clin Oral Implants Res 2004;15(1):82–95.

45. Chiapasco M, Zaniboni M, Rimondini L. Autogenous onlay bone grafts vs. alveolar distraction osteogenesis for the correction of vertically deficient edentulous ridges: a 2–4-year prospective study on humans. Clin Oral Implants Res 2007;18(4):432–40.

46. Uckan S, Veziroglu F, Dayangac E. Alveolar distraction osteogenesis versus autogenous onlay bone grafting for alveolar ridge augmentation: technique, complications, and implant survival rates. Oral Surg Oral Med Oral Pathol Oral Radiol Endod 2008;106(4):511–5.

47. Bianchi A, Felice P, Lizio G, et al. Alveolar distraction osteogenesis versus inlay bone grafting in posterior mandibular atrophy: a prospective study. Oral Surg Oral Med Oral Pathol Oral Radiol Endod 2008; 105(3):282–92.

48. Chiapasco M, Zaniboni M, Boisco M. Augmentation procedures for the rehabilitation of deficient edentulous ridges with oral implants. Clin Oral Implants Res 2006;17(Suppl 2):136–59.

49. Alkan A, Baş B, Inal S. Alveolar distraction osteogenesis of bone graft reconstructed mandible. Oral Surg Oral Med Oral Pathol Oral Radiol Endod 2005;100(3):e39–42.

50. Kunkel M, Wahlmann U, Reichert TE, et al. Reconstruction of mandibular defects following tumor ablation by vertical distraction osteogenesis using intraosseous distraction devices. Clin Oral Implants Res 2005;16(1):89–97.

51. Hirota M, Mizuki N, Iwai T, et al. Vertical distraction of a free vascularized osteocutaneous scapular flap in the reconstructed mandible for implant therapy. Int J Oral Maxillofac Surg 2008;37(5):481–3.

52. Hirota M, Matsui Y, Mizuki N, et al. Management considerations in reconstruction of postablative defects of the mandible: vertical distraction of a scapular bone flap and removable lip support: a case report. Oral Surg Oral Med Oral Pathol Oral Radiol Endod 2008;106(6):e6–9.

53. Levin L, Carrasco L, Kazemi A, et al. Enhancement of the fibula free flap by alveolar distraction for dental implant restoration: report of a case. Facial Plast Surg 2003;19(1):87–94.

54. Lizio G, Corinaldesi G, Pieri F, et al. Problems with dental implants that were placed on vertically distracted fibular free flaps after resection: a report of six cases. Br J Oral Maxillofac Surg 2009;47(6):455–60.

55. Chiapasco M, Consolo U, Bianchi A, et al. Alveolar distraction osteogenesis for the correction of vertically deficient edentulous ridges: a multicenter prospective study on humans. Int J Oral Maxillofac Implants 2004;19(3):399–407.

56. Raghoebar GM, Stellingsma K, Meijer HJ, et al. Vertical distraction of the severely resorbed edentulous mandible: an assessment of treatment outcome. Int J Oral Maxillofac Implants 2008;23(2):299–307.

57. Elo JA, Herford AS, Boyne PJ. Implant success in distracted bone versus autogenous bone-grafted sites. J Oral Implantol 2009;35(4):181–4.

58. Polo WC, de Araujo NS, Lima YB, et al. Peri-implant bone loss around posterior mandible dental implants placed after distraction osteogenesis: preliminary findings. J Periodontol 2007;78(2):204–8.

59. Degidi M, Pieri F, Marchetti C, et al. Immediate loading of dental implants placed in distracted bone: a case report. Int J Oral Maxillofac Implants 2004;19(3):448–54.

60. Bilbao A, Oliveira MH, Varela-Centelles PI, et al. Assessment of dental implant stability in osseo-distraction-generated bone: a resonance frequency analysis. Clin Oral Implants Res 2009; 20(8):772–7.

61. Robiony M, Zorzan E, Polini F, et al. Osteogenesis distraction and platelet-rich plasma: combined use in restoration of severe atrophic mandible. Long-term results. Clin Oral Implants Res 2008;19(11):1202–10.

62. Schortinghuis J, Bronckers AL, Gravendeel J, et al. The effect of ultrasound on osteogenesis in the vertically distracted edentulous mandible: a double-blind trial. Int J Oral Maxillofac Surg 2008;37(11):1014–21.

63. Dergin G, Gurler G, Guvercin M, et al. Vertical alveolar bone distraction with polytetrafloroethylene membrane for implant application: a technical note. J Oral Maxillofac Surg 2007;65(5):1050–4.

64. Allais M, Maurette PE, Mazzonetto R, et al. Patient's perception of the events during and after osteogenic alveolar distraction. Med Oral Patol Oral Cir Bucal 2007;12(3):E225–8.

65. Castry G, Ella B, Emparanza A, et al. Impact psychologique de la distraction alvéolaire mandibulaire [Psychological impact of alveolar mandibular distraction]. Rev Stomatol Chir Maxillofac 2009; 110(5):251–5 [in French].

66. Enislidis G, Fock N, Ewers R. Distraction osteogenesis with subperiosteal devices in edentulous mandibles. Br J Oral Maxillofac Surg 2005;43(5): 399–403.

67. Mazzonetto R, Allais M, Maurette PE, et al. A retrospective study of the potential complications during alveolar distraction osteogenesis in 55 patients. Int J Oral Maxillofac Surg 2007;36(1):6–10.

68. Saulacić N, Somosa Martín M, de Los Angeles Leon Camacho M, et al. Complications in alveolar distraction osteogenesis: a clinical investigation. J Oral Maxillofac Surg 2007;65(2):267–74.

69. Perdijk FB, Meijer GJ, Strijen PJ, et al. Complications in alveolar distraction osteogenesis of the atrophic mandible. Int J Oral Maxillofac Surg 2007;36(10): 916–21.

70. Günbay T, Koyuncu BO, Akay MC, et al. Results and complications of alveolar distraction osteogenesis to enhance vertical bone height. Oral Surg Oral Med Oral Pathol Oral Radiol Endod 2008;105(5):e7–13.

71. Saulacic N, Zix J, Iizuka T. Complication rates and associated factors in alveolar distraction osteogenesis: a comprehensive review. Int J Oral Maxillofac Surg 2009;38(3):210–7.

Soft Tissue Considerations in Implant Site Development

Nicolaas C. Geurs, DDS, MS, Philip J. Vassilopoulos, DDS,
Michael S. Reddy, DMD, DMSc*

KEYWORDS

• Soft-tissue • Regeneration • Prosthesis • Implant therapy

THE CHARACTERISTICS OF SOFT TISSUE SURROUNDING IMPLANTS

Healthy soft tissue surrounding a dental implant is essential for successful implant restoration. This success includes the establishment of health, function, and esthetics. The functional implant restoration must have a component that traverses the oral mucosa. As with a natural tooth, there is a need to provide a connection or seal around the neck of the implant or an abutment. The development process of the tooth includes the formation of a biologic connection between the living tissues. For a dental implant, this connection has to be created during the healing process after placement of the implant; the difference being that the oral mucosa will have to interface with a foreign body. The resulting attachment, although similar in function, has biologic differences that must be comprehended to design surgical techniques and biomaterials that will surround the dental implant with biologically functional and esthetic soft tissue. The success of dental implants is dependent on the establishment of a soft-tissue barrier that is able to shelter the underlying osseous structures and the osseointegration surrounding the implant body. The esthetics of a dental implant prosthesis depend on the health and stability of the peri-implant mucosa. Understanding of soft-tissue healing and maintenance around dental implants is paramount for implant success. This article discusses the soft-tissue interface, aspects of soft-tissue health, and esthetics during treatment planning and therapy.

THE SOFT-TISSUE INTERFACE

Bone grafting as part of the site development will be less successful without healthy soft tissue overlying the osseous graft. The implant–soft-tissue-bone interface is similar to that of natural teeth. The function of the epithelium surrounding dental implants is similar to gingival epithelium. It includes an oral epithelium, a sulcular epithelium, and a junctional epithelium with underlying connective tissue. From the gingival margin into the sulcus the epithelium changes to sulcular epithelium and ends in a junctional or barrier epithelium.[1–3] This junctional barrier protects the bone supporting the tooth. When the mucosal wound is created to place the implant or attach the abutment, the surrounding epithelium will migrate over the fibrin clot or granulation tissue. Once the epithelium reaches the implant surface, migration will occur in an apical direction. Despite being in contact with the implant surface during apical proliferation, the epithelium will undergo major morphologic and functional changes and the junctional epithelium will be formed. The attachment is facilitated by the basal lamina and the formation of hemidesmosomes.[4,5] The epithelial downgrowth is believed to be limited by the presence of underlying granulation tissue.

Department of Periodontology, University of Alabama at Birmingham, 1530 Third Avenue South, SDB 412, Birmingham, AL 35294-0007, USA
* Corresponding author.
E-mail address: mreddy@uab.edu

Oral Maxillofacial Surg Clin N Am 22 (2010) 387–405
doi:10.1016/j.coms.2010.04.001
1042-3699/10/$ – see front matter. Published by Elsevier Inc.

Adhesion of this connective tissue to the implant will prevent the apical movement of the epithelium. As the maturity of the connective tissue increases around the implant it will limit the epithelial apical migration.[6,7] Berglundh and colleagues[1] hypothesized that contact with the titanium oxide layer would prevent epithelial downgrowth. The implant surface characteristics can also influence apical migration of epithelium.[8] The epithelial attachment can be observed after 1 to 2 weeks of healing, and a mature barrier epithelium occurs after 6 to 8 weeks of healing.[3] The ability of biomaterials to promote epithelial wound healing and to establish a junctional epithelium is an important aspect of the success of dental implant bone site preparation. The protection of the connective tissue and osseous tissue surrounding the implant by providing this barrier is crucial for the maintenance of peri-implant structures and the stability of the implant system. Poor gingival health and chronic inflammation will compromise this process.

The apical portion of the junctional epithelium is separated from the alveolar crest by a zone of connective tissue.[9] This is where the similarities between the natural tooth and the implant soft tissues end. During healing, the adhesion of the fibrin clot results in the formation of granulation tissue. Collagen fibers of the mucosa are organized after 4 to 6 weeks of healing.[3] The connective tissue is void of fibroblast and vascular structures and rich in fibers. It resembles scar tissue and is an important part of the seal that forms around the implant surface to exclude the oral environment.[2,10–12]

The dentogingival fibers around a natural tooth insert into cementum and bone and are firmly attached. These fibers serve as a barrier of epithelial downgrowth and are important for the seal function of the gingiva.[11] The dental implant surface does not contain a layer of cementum, therefore the fibers do not insert into the titanium surface of the implant. Collagen fibers surrounding the dental implant surface form a cuff. The connective tissue adhesion at the implant has less mechanical resistance than that of natural teeth.[12,13]

Surface characteristics of the implant influence the orientation of the fibers, which are mostly parallel to the implant surface when the implant surface is smooth.[1,6,14] Surface roughness provides for different stimulation, allowing connective tissue to be embedded into the surface. When implants are loaded, the orientation of these fibers is more traverse.[15,16] The orientation of the collagen fibers is more perpendicular to the surface in implants with a roughened surface interface in the soft connective tissue zone.[17] In a human histologic and scanning electron microscope (SEM) evaluation of soft tissue surrounding 2-piece implants with laser microgrooved channels, fibers were found in close contact with the microgrooves and were oriented perpendicular to the implant surface, showing more similarities to natural dentition.[8] The fibroblast-rich layer adjacent to the titanium surface has an important role in the maintenance of a proper seal between the oral environment and the peri-implant tissue.[18] The quality of the mucosal barrier depends on the material of the surface. In an animal experiment, mucosal healing with a zone of connective tissue attachment was observed around titanium and ceramic abutments but not around gold alloys.[19]

Collagen type V, which has a higher collagenase stability, was localized in higher amounts in the lamina propria of the peri-implant gingival tissues, as compared to natural teeth. This anatomic difference may be responsible for the defense of peri-implant keratinized gingival connective tissues to bacterial penetration.[20]

THE VASCULAR SUPPLY OF THE PERI-IMPLANT MUCOSA

The main vascular supply for the gingiva is derived from the supraperiosteal blood vessels and the anastomosis with the vessels from the periodontal ligament and alveolar bone. The vascular supply of the peri-implant mucosa is almost solely supplied by the supraperiosteal blood vessels. An osseointegrated implant does not have a periodontal ligament, and therefore the blood supply is markedly different from the situation around a tooth. During the osseogenesis phase, bone surrounding the implant undergoes osseoconduction, de novo bone, and remodeling resulting in osseointegration. The bone surrounding an implant has increased density and is void of vessels.[21,22] When a thin layer of bone is present surrounding an implant, infraosseous vessels diminish or disappear. Remodeling following extraction could result in diminished dimensions of the remaining bone.[23] When implants are placed in close proximity to a natural tooth or to another implant, the dimensions of the osseous tissue bone are reduced and the vascular supply compromised. The lack of anastamosis reduces the blood supply to the peri-implant connective tissue.[2,10–12] Understanding the differences in the vascular supply and the importance of angiogenesis and the vascular supply to wound healing are important for the design of surgical techniques.

KERATINIZED ATTACHED MUCOSA

The stability of the peri-implant mucosa is important for the overall stability of the dental implant and the maintenance of bone health around an implant. Whether the stability is secured by non-keratinized mucosa or keratinized attached mucosa is a point of discussion. Some investigators report no difference in the maintenance of peri-implant bone levels,[24–26] whereas others report an increased risk for peri-implant bone loss when the implant is surrounded by alveolar mucosa.[27,28] Insufficient keratinized mucosa in the vicinity of implants does not necessarily mediate adverse effects on hygiene management.[24]

The lack of consensus regarding peri-implant soft-tissue health is related to multifactorial issues. Oral hygiene, host immunologic responses, implant design, location in the mouth, local anatomy, function, and surgical techniques make it difficult to design studies that will give conclusive answers.

The advantages of keratinized attached mucosa surrounding the implant are less controversial. Most clinicians prefer to surround the implant with an adequate zone of keratinized mucosa. The advantages include the overall health of the tissues, greater patient satisfaction, and fewer complications.[28]

The stability of the mucosa will provide better support for the underlying connective tissue, and the junctional epithelium will provide the seal around the implant. As a result of the increased stability of the tissues, prosthetic techniques are more precise. Challenges to the soft tissue during the prosthodontic phase are better absorbed by keratinized tissue.[10,25,26]

When considering the final esthetics, a wide band of keratinized mucosa is a prerequisite.[29,30] A thick biotype offers the ability to hide the shine-through of the underlying structures.[26,31]

THE BIOLOGIC WIDTH

The dimensions of the physiologic dentogingival junction around natural teeth is referred to as the biologic width. It encompasses the width of the epithelial and connective attachments when evaluated with histology. In a classic report using cadaver specimens, the average width of the epithelial attachment was 1.07 mm, connective tissue attachment 0.97 mm with an average biologic width of 2.04 mm around the natural tooth.[32] These measurements are averages, and individual differences exist, based on the location in the mouth and aspect of the tooth.[33,34] The greatest variation was found in the epithelial attachment,

whereas the connective tissue attachment varied the least.[35] The biologic width represents the zone responsible for the establishment of the dentogingival junction and the seal around the tooth. Violation of the biologic width will result in a disruption of the seal function, which becomes evident when the margin of a restoration is placed within the zone of the soft-tissue attachment and disrupts the dentogingival junction.[36]

The earlier outline of an epithelial attachment and a connective tissue attachment to the implant surface showed the similarities between the attachment around a tooth and an implant. The establishment of this zone of biologic width around an implant has been found around nonsubmerged and 2-piece submerged implants.[2,10,37–39] Around a nonsubmerged implant, the biologic width establishes itself in the months following implant placement.[3] Once established, the dimensions of biologic width are stable[38] and are not influenced if implants are loaded early.[40] The dimensions are approximately 2 mm for the epithelial attachment and 1 mm for the connective tissue attachment. This will guide the surgeon's decision for pre-implant bone grafting.

One-piece nonsubmerged implant systems offer several advantages, including the need for only 1 surgery, a mature soft-tissue implant interface, and avoidance of a microgap.[41] For 2-piece implant systems, a zone of attachment is formed after placement of an abutment. In an animal model, soft-tissue height around a 2-piece implant was reduced at abutment attachment to less than 2 mm.[42] Compared with a control with no reduction, the soft-tissue levels were lower; however, the zone of biologic width was the same after 6 months. The implants with thinned soft tissue showed bone resorption around the neck of the implant accounting for the re-establishment of a zone of attachment or biologic width around an implant. Peri-implant bone remodeling could be influenced by the establishment of the biologic width.[10] The bone resorption around the implant neck does not start until the implant is uncovered and exposed to the oral cavity. The bacterial contamination of the gap between the implant and the superstructure is one of the factors influencing crestal bone loss.[13,43–48]

The loss is in height, but there is also a horizontal component that has greater consequences when implants are placed adjacent to one another. The zone of bone loss in a horizontal direction could overlap and result in loss of interimplant bone height, and with it the interimplant papillary height. This problem is an issue when implants are placed closer than 3 mm apart.[44] The dimensions of the biologic width are stable in a well-healed 2-piece implant without additional challenges.[37] The dimensions of the biologic width around an implant are implant-system specific. In an animal model, implants of different configurations were placed in varying locations in relation to the crest of the bone. The biologic width dimension for 1-piece implants, with the rough/smooth border located at the bone crest level, were smaller compared with 2-piece implants with a microgap located at or below the crest of the bone. Biologic width dimensions are more similar to natural teeth around 1-piece nonsubmerged implants compared with 2-piece nonsubmerged or 2-piece submerged implants. The location of the microgap has an influence on bone maintenance and soft-tissue attachment. When the microgap is placed below the crest, remodeling of the bone results in bone loss apical to the crest. The connective tissue attachment is on the implant surface and bone is never found coronal to the microgap. Bone was not found on a machined surface but always on the roughened surface. The size of the microgap did not influence the amount of bone loss. The micromobility of the abutment connection also resulted in greater amounts of bone remodeling.[39,45] When the microgap is placed below the crest, greater amounts of inflammation were present surrounding the neck of the implant, resulting in greater bone loss.[46,47]

With submerged implants, early spontaneous exposure results in crestal bone loss.[48] Small exposures not exposing the full cover screw are associated with greater amounts of bone loss.[49] When spontaneous exposure occurs, it is recommended to expose the implant completely.[50]

The issue of bone healing and maintenance around the cervical portion is an area of debate. Many factors are discussed as having an influence on bone stability. During the surgical procedure, trauma may occur and result in loss of the crestal bone during healing. It is important to follow proper surgical protocols to minimize trauma or overheating. The flap design may also be influential on the amount of initial bone loss. In an animal experiment, less bone loss was found using a flapless approach after 3 months of healing.[51] The implant surface characteristics are also important. Bone loss around implants when the junction between a smooth and roughened surface was placed apical to the crest of bone occurred to the level of the roughened surface.[39,45]

Most of the literature regarding biologic width around dental implants concerns implants with a machined portion of the implant that has been the designated area of soft-tissue attachment. This situation was established at the time of implant placement or at the time of the second-stage surgery followed by bone remodeling.

Some implants have a roughness that extends to the collar of the implant. This roughness provides better support of the implant but could also enhance biofilm formation.[52] Surface tension on the implant surface can also enhance the formation and attachment of a biofilm.[53] Some implant designs use a beveled collar or even a horizontal part of the implant platform for the soft-tissue attachment. The dimensions of the attachment are similar, but the height of soft tissue coronal to the crest of bone can be reduced.[54] This concept has been shown to reduce the amount of crestal bone loss.[55,56] Implant surfaces that facilitate the attachment of the soft tissues can also result in more stability of the soft-tissue zone around an implant.[8]

Schwarz and colleagues[17] evaluated histologic sections of a healed implant with high hydrophilicity and a microtopography. They concluded that soft-tissue integration is enhanced on surfaces with increased surface tension.

Implants with microgrooved laser etched collars resulted in less crestal bone loss compared with control implants without the microgrooves. The use of tissue-engineered collars with microgrooving seems to promote bone and soft-tissue attachment along the collar and facilitate development of a biologic width, and seems not to lead to an increase in biofilm on the implant surfaces.[57,58]

OSSEOUS SUPPORT FOR SOFT TISSUES

Thus far, this article has emphasized soft-tissue attachment to the implant surface and stabilizing of the implant by protecting the bone. However, the reverse relationship is also true. The lack of proper bone volume surrounding a dental implant will result in the loss of peri-implant bone and the loss of soft-tissue height or recession around a dental implant. This outcome is important in planning for an implant. It is important to understand the importance of site development because of the support that hard tissue gives to soft tissue. Bone support is important for the presence of a papilla around an implant restoration.

THE PAPILLA AROUND IMPLANT RESTORATIONS

The interdental papilla is an important aspect of the esthetic appearance of a smile. The lack of the dental papilla results in a dark triangle that will make the esthetics less desirable. The presence of the papilla between natural teeth is dependent on the presence of 2 adjacent teeth, a contact point, and supporting bone. If the crest of the bone is within 5 mm of the contact point, the full presence of a papilla is predictable. If the distance increases, the likelihood of the papilla being present decreases.[59] A similar relationship has been reported around dental implants. The important measurement is the level of the bone on the proximal surface of the adjacent tooth. On restorations with papillae, the average distance to the crest of bone is slightly reduced compared with that of natural teeth.[60–66] The attachment on the adjacent tooth provides for the support of the papilla.[61] The situation between dental implants is different. The interimplant is supported by 2 implant surfaces. As discussed earlier, the soft tissue lacks the insertion of fibers. There is potential for overlapping crestal resorption if the implants are placed too close together. Implants placed closer than 3 mm to each other exhibit greater amounts of bone loss.[44] The height of the interimplant papilla is limited and, in general, no greater than 3 mm from the underlying bone.[62,63] In the esthetic areas, the results may be improved by avoiding 2 dental implants adjacent to each other or choosing implants of a smaller diameter to ensure a minimum of 3 mm between the implants.[63] In areas of limited space, small-diameter implants could be considered. The smaller diameter leaves a greater space for soft tissues and provides a created osseous base for the support of soft tissues around an implant.[64]

IMPLANT PLANNING FOR OPTIMAL SOFT-TISSUE OUTCOMES
The Edentulous Patient

In fully edentulous patients, soft-tissue evaluation should include a soft-tissue–specific clinical examination to assess the condition of soft tissue and to investigate the presence of keratinized mucosa.[65]

The conflicting evidence on the necessity of keratinized and attached mucosa surrounding dental implants for optimal outcomes must be addressed before proceeding with soft-tissue evaluation. In an animal study, the lack of keratinized peri-implant mucosa and accumulated plaque resulted in soft-tissue recession.[66] In a human study, 58 patients received 307 implants for a full-arch, fixed mandibular prosthesis.[67] A lack of peri-implant keratinized mucosa was associated with buccal soft-tissue recession as well as lingual plaque accumulation and bleeding. There was no correlation of the buccal plaque accumulation and bleeding with the subjects who had peri-implant keratinized mucosa.

In another human study, Wennström and colleagues[68] evaluated the influence of the width of keratinized mucosa on the maintenance of peri-implant soft-tissue health in complete

dentures and fixed partial-denture reconstruction cases. These findings differed from the previous ones; in this study 24% of sites lacked keratinized mucosa, 13% of sites had less than 2 mm of keratinized mucosa, and 61% of sites exhibited mobility of soft-tissue margins around the implants. The author concluded that there was no effect on the mobility of the marginal peri-implant soft tissue and the absence of keratinized mucosa had no impact. Hence, the health of peri-implant tissues, as determined by bleeding on probing, shows that a lack of keratinized mucosa does not clearly indicate inevitable recession.

Clinically, implant insertion within the keratinized mucosa is preferred. The level of oral hygiene and inflammation rather than keratinized mucosa is the predominant determinant of soft-tissue health around an implant.

The Partially Edentulous Patient

In implant dentistry, esthetics are a significant consideration for the dentate population. The gingival scaffold frames the shape of the implant restoration and is important for simulation of the natural dentition.[69]

The treatment planning of edentulous spaces in the esthetic zone presents surgical and restorative challenges. Soft-tissue examination before implant procedures is of great importance in determining the predictability of a treatment approach.

Kopp and Belser[70] proposed a series of objective criteria relating to dental esthetics. The evaluation of a tooth-bound edentulous site should include periodontal examination and probing, ridge mapping, bone sounding, and gingival biotype.

When a tooth needs to be extracted and is to be replaced by a dental implant, the implant site soft-tissue evaluation begins with the clinical examination of periodontal status of the specific tooth and the adjacent teeth. Periodontal probing will determine the periodontal attachment levels of these teeth and will identify any existing pathology. Probing should be complemented by periapical radiographs that reveal the interproximal bone levels of the adjacent teeth.

The attachment levels of the adjacent teeth are the predetermining factor for the level of interproximal bone and soft-tissue height. For an edentulous site, the assessment may require ridge mapping.[71] Mapping entails a series of soft-tissue thickness buccal and lingual measurements of the area. The clinician can then transfer these measurements onto a cast by taking an impression of this area, pouring a diagnostic cast, sectioning the cast through the proposed implant site, and transferring the soft-tissue thickness around the alveolar crest. Information related to the soft-tissue profile, the underlying bone morphology, and bone dimensions is readily available in the cast and could be of use for the clinician when determining the need for bone grafting or even additional soft-tissue grafting of the implant site. Although cone beam computed tomography may provide more accurate and detailed information about implant sites, bone mapping of a single-tooth edentulous area is a quick and inexpensive method of assessing bone and soft-tissue volume.

Bone sounding is a technique-sensitive procedure that detects the height of bone at the cervical region of a hopeless tooth. The accuracy and successful outcome in using this technique is based on a clinician's experience and accurate measurements of anatomic variations such as tooth crown morphology and thickness of the alveolar crest. Bone sounding is best used to examine soft tissue around a tooth that will be extracted and immediately replaced by an implant.

The soft-tissue examination should include the assessment of the gingival biotype of the implant site and adjacent teeth. This type of evaluation is particularly useful in immediate implant situations. Thin and thick biotypes are characteristically different (**Fig. 1**). A thin gingival biotype is characterized by high-scalloped thin soft tissue, slender teeth, and long interproximal gingival embrasure spaces with small contact points located at the incisal third of the teeth. There is a strong correlation of thin biotype with the presence of bone

fenestrations and dehiscence. Moreover, a thin biotype is susceptible to soft-tissue recession after surgical procedures. Conversely, a thick gingival biotype has a low-scalloped thick soft tissue, square teeth, and small gingival embrasure spaces, and long contact surfaces positioned at the middle third of the teeth. This biotype is more resistant to recession after surgical manipulation of soft tissue.[72–75]

Immediate implant placement in a thin-tissue biotype is associated with high risk of experiencing soft-tissue recession, as opposed to patients with a thick-tissue biotype.

DIAGNOSIS AND CLASSIFICATION

A series of classification systems has been developed to address soft- and hard-tissue deformities of edentulous ridges before implant surgery. These classifications provide the clinician with specific guidelines to proceed in assembling an appropriate treatment plan. The classification of sites may be helpful in forecasting the outcome of bone and soft-tissue grafting procedures to achieve successful function and esthetics.

Seibert[76] proposed the following classification for edentulous ridge soft-tissue defects:

1. Class I: soft-tissue deformity of the edentulous ridge in a buccolingual dimension
2. Class II: soft-tissue deformity of the edentulous ridge in an apicocoronal dimension

A

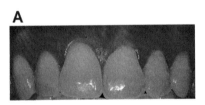

B

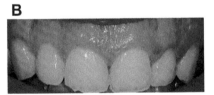

Delicate thin gingiva	Dense, more fibrotic keratinized gingiva
Osseous form scalloped and thin	Osseous form flatter and thicker
Dehiscence and fenestrations likely	
Small amount of attached keratinized gingiva	Larger amount of attached keratinized gingiva
Scalloped shape	Flat shape
Reacts to insult with recession	Reacts to insult in pocket formation Recession not likely
Papilla to cervical margin distance greater	Papilla to cervical margin distance smaller
Contact point in incisal third	Contac point more apical
Teeth triangular in shape	Teeth square in shape

Fig. 1. (*A*) Thin scalloped periodontal biotype. (*B*) Thick flat periodontal biotype.

3. Class III: soft-tissue deformity of the edentulous ridge in both dimensions.

Palacci and Nowzari[77] developed a classification system combining soft- and hard-tissue defects. Greater challenges for reconstruction of the underlying hard tissue supporting the soft tissue exist for defects that have a vertical component.

Jemt[61] conducted a retrospective study in 21 patients with 25 single-implant crowns. He evaluated the papillary height of soft tissue between single-implant crowns and teeth and created an index for assessment of soft-tissue contours around implants.

The Jemt index comprises 5 different scores:

1. Index score 0: absence of papilla
2. Index score 1: less than half of the papilla present
3. Index score 2: more than half of the papilla present but not reaching the contact point between the implant crown and the adjacent tooth
4. Index score 3: the papilla fills the entire embrasure space
5. Index score 4: the papilla is enlarged and overfills the interproximal space.

Esthetic compromises occur when the papilla does not completely fill the interproximal space under the contact point, resulting in the display of a black triangle. This condition is consistent with Jemt index 0 to 2 and is difficult to correct.

Implant Placement

Optimal implant position should consider the three-dimensional placement of implants that respects established biologic and prosthetic principles related to implant restoration. The relationship between the bone and the implant determines the dental implant soft-tissue contours, including interproximal papilla. The relationship defines the esthetic appearance of the final implant prosthesis. A successful outcome is maintained for a period of time because it preserves the original soft-tissue morphology and features.

Specific placement guidelines have been developed to accomplish soft-tissue stability around dental implants. These guidelines are applicable when bone is sufficient and of good quality:

1. The apicocoronal placement of the dental implant platform should be positioned 3 mm below the facial marginal tissue (**Fig. 2**).[78] The 3-mm rule was created for the following reasons:

- The 3-mm space is needed on the prosthetic abutment for formation of biologic width
- An ideal emergence profile of implant restorations needs room for a smooth transition from the circular implant platform to the triangular or square abutment and crown
- There is room available for placement of restorative margins below marginal soft tissue
- The possibility of peri-implant marginal soft-tissue recession is more likely as the patient ages

2. Buccolingually, the implant is placed so that the outer aspect of its platform is 1 mm palatal from the anticipated facial margins of the restoration. Some clinicians use a 2-mm placement rule from the facial cortical plate in anticipation of the 1.4-mm lateral bone loss as a guideline.[79] Kan and Rungcharassaeng[80] recommended that the buccolingual placement be 1 mm palatal in relation to facial emergence profiles of the adjacent teeth, and not less than 1 mm because of the risk of losing the facial bone and soft tissue

3. The implant platform is located on the same axis with the gingival zenith and 3 mm lower than the free soft-tissue margin. Magne and Belser[81] suggested that the gingival zenith is distal to the long axis of maxillary anterior teeth. Although Rufenacht[82] noted that the gingival zenith of lateral incisors is in the same line as their long axis, and that only central and lateral incisors have the gingival zenith on the distal third of the tooth (**Fig. 3**).

IMPLANT SPACING

Spacing requirements between tooth and implant, as well as spacing between implants, were developed to preserve the bone and overlying soft-tissue support of the implant and crown.

The minimum recommended distance between a tooth and an implant is 1.5 mm, based on a study by Esposito and colleagues.[83] The study indicated a strong correlation between bone loss of adjacent teeth and horizontal distance of the implant fixture to the tooth. The greatest amount of bone loss was noted at the lateral incisor position. Although all the implant fixtures were 4.1 mm in diameter, and bone loss increased as the distance was decreased, only 17% of bone loss variation was attributed to this reduced distance. It seems that other intra- and interindividual parameters played a role.

The minimum recommended interimplant distance is 3 mm in a 2-stage implant protocol.

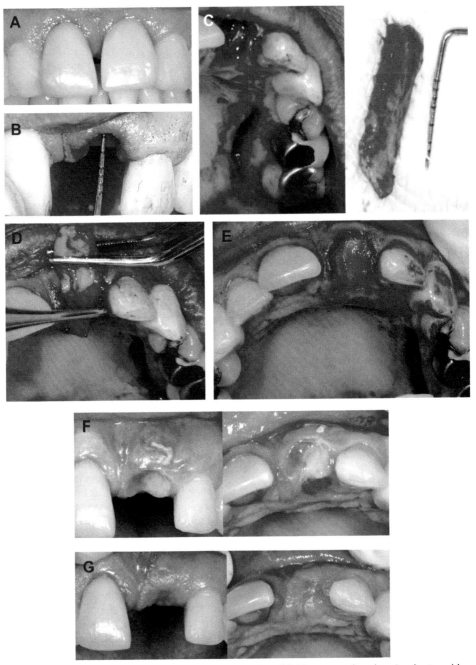

Fig. 2. Fig. 2. (*A*) Gingival height around #9 prior to extraction. (*B*) #9 extracted and an implant and bone graft placed; tip of probe placed on top of platform of implant. (*C*) Sub-epithelial connective tissue graft harvested from the palate. (*D*) CT graft placed in a pouch on the palatal and facial aspect. (*E*) CT graft covers the implant and graft. (*F*) Soft tissue healing at 2 weeks. (*G*) Soft tissue healing after 2 months.

Tarnow and colleagues[44] conducted a retrospective radiographic study in 36 patients who had 2 adjacent implants placed. The author found that lateral bone loss at the implant-abutment interface was 1.34 to 1.4 mm. This finding had an effect on the height of bone and papilla support between implants within a distance of less than 3 mm. When implants were within 3 mm of each other, they developed 1.04 mm of interproximal bone loss compared with 0.45 mm of bone loss for the implants placed with more than 3 mm distance between them.

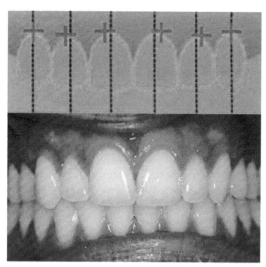

Fig. 3. The location of the gingival zenith. + Indicates the location of the gingival zenith located distal to the long axis of the maxillary incisors.

Based on the potential for interproximal bone loss on adjacent implants, Grunder and colleagues[79] proposed buccal augmentation of the site in situations with less than 3 mm of bone interproximally. They proposed that the bone thickness should be augmented to at least 2 mm, and ideally 4 mm, to maintain the soft-tissue height facially and interproximally. The investigators suggested that the additional bone can support and maintain the interproximal papilla.

The three-dimensional implant placement guidelines and spacing requirements may lead to the use of small-diameter implants in the esthetic zone that allow bone preservation between implants as well as between implant and tooth. The narrow diameter implants may provide more bone support in all dimensions for development of the soft-tissue form that simulates the natural dentition.[64]

SURGICAL AUGMENTATION OF SOFT TISSUE AROUND DENTAL IMPLANTS

Peri-implant soft-tissue management can be regarded as a category of mucogingival procedures analogous to reconstructive procedures around teeth including root coverage, papilla reconstruction, ridge augmentation, and ridge preservation. These soft-tissue augmentation procedures can be accomplished at the time of extraction before implant placement, at implant placement, at the time the implant is uncovered, or even after the completed restoration has been placed.[84]

Although the ability to permanently replace single or multiple missing teeth with osseointegrated dental implants has been thoroughly reported in the literature, with consistent long-term results,[85–93] dental implant therapy can be complicated by numerous developmental, traumatic, or anatomic factors such as a thin gingival biotype in association with a high smile line, leading to esthetic shortcomings in the anterior maxilla. Therefore, various soft-tissue augmentation techniques have been advocated to provide better esthetic outcomes.[86,87] These studies have proposed procedures used to treat dehiscence defects, achieve primary soft-tissue closure over single implants immediately placed into maxillary extraction sockets (with or without guided bone regeneration), and improve soft-tissue healing.

SURGICAL TECHNIQUES FOR AUGMENTATION
Pedicle Grafts

Pedicle full- or split-thickness palatal flaps for primary coverage of implants placed after extraction and treatment of maxillary peri-implant defects have been described in numerous reports in the literature.

Nemcovsky and colleagues[88] described a rotated split palatal flap (RSPF) technique for soft-tissue primary coverage over extraction sites with immediate implant placement. This technique was used only if palatal mucosal thickness exceeded 4 mm. The surgical procedure consisted of a full-thickness mucoperiosteal palatal flap that was raised, extending at least 1 tooth mesially and distally from the tooth to be extracted. A minimal buccal flap, including only interdental papillae and marginal gingiva, exposing the bone crest, was also reflected. The tooth was carefully extracted and the implant was placed slightly palatal and off center. The palatal flap was split into deep and superficial layers. A second incision, involving only the deeper flap, further disconnected these 2 flaps. The deeper flap was thus transformed into a pediculated flap, becoming mobile and easily rotated. The RSPF was tucked and sutured under the minimally reflected buccal flap, covering the implant site. The superficial layer of the palatal flap was then repositioned and sutured. Consequently, complete primary soft-tissue closure over the implant site was achieved. This technique is sometimes used to change the gingival thickness in an edentulous space (**Fig. 4**).

One year later, Nemcovsky and colleagues[89] proposed the use of full-thickness rotated palatal flap (RPF) only when palatal gingival thickness measures 5 mm or less at the time of immediate implant placement after extraction of maxillary anterior and premolar teeth. In this case, a sharp, deep, internal-beveled incision delineating a pediculated full-thickness palatal flap was made. The extension was planned to enable full coverage of the alveolus and overlapping of the buccal crestal bone, usually extending 1 or 2 proximal teeth on both sides. The pediculated flap was then carefully elevated from the underlying bone, starting from the side away from the tooth. An oblique proximal incision and periosteal fenestration facilitated rotation of the pediculated flap, which was wider than 5 mm. Buccal margins of the RPF were de-epithelialized. The pediculated flap was then rotated with the use of atraumatic surgical pliers, tucked, and sutured under the reflected minimal buccal flap. Further sutures secured the RPF in the palatal tissues. The donor palatal site, which was left exposed, healed by secondary intention.

Conversely, the palatal subepithelial connective tissue flap method to cover maxillary defects was promoted by Khoury and Happe.[90] According to this technique, a palatal paramarginal incision was made from the molar region to the defect to be covered. The length of the incision depended on the size of the defect. Dissection of the muco-periosteal flap and the underlying preparation of a subepithelial connective tissue flap to a depth of 5 to 8 mm were then performed. A sharp incision of the subepithelial tissue was made parallel to the first incision in the same manner to harvest a connective tissue graft, but leaving it attached in the anterior region. The subepithelial connective tissue flap was elevated and rotated to cover the defect or reconstruct soft tissue. Because the donor site is situated in a well-vascularized area (palatal artery), heavy bleeding can occur and may require cauterization. Because only a subepithelial connective tissue flap was removed, the palatal wound at the donor site could be totally closed and sutured.

Goldstein and colleagues[87] described the palatal advanced flap technique for single-implant and multiple-implant cases, with the same efficiency and with highly predictable results. First, the mesiodistal, and especially the labiopalatal, aspects of the gap were measured. Then, the outline of an L-shaped flap with parallel incisions was marked. The flap was planned so that the long leg of the L was toward the distal and the short leg was perpendicular to the extraction site. The distance between the parallel incisions had to be equal to the mesiodistal size of the extraction site. A triangular area was marked coronal to the incisions, in the inner part of the L-shaped flap. The base of the triangle was on the short leg of the L, and its apex was pointed distally along the long leg. This arrangement was the key part of this technique, and careful planning was required so that the base of the triangle was equal in size to the labiopalatal dimension of the gap area. The dimensions of the triangle area determined the amount of coronal advancement of the flap. At this stage, the triangular area was de-epithelialized, and the L-shaped area was dissected, performing a split-thickness dissection. The flap was advanced in a coronal position and sutured with 6-0 or 5-0 sutures. Thus, complete and precise coverage of the implant area was achieved without any tension. A denuded area was left on the apical side of the flap.

Free Gingival Grafts

Free gingival grafts have been used to correct or limit the potential for soft-tissue complications around endosseous implant permucosal abutments. The rationale for free gingival grafting is largely to prevent peri-implantitis and its associated bone loss by increasing the amount of keratinized mucosa adjacent to the implant abutment.[91] This approach is believed to have 2 potential benefits. First, keratinized tissue is believed to form a more stable seal on a smooth titanium or zirconium abutment, limiting the potential for biofilm migration down to the implant interface. Second, keratinized tissue is generally firmer and less subject to abrasion from tooth brushing and other oral hygiene practices, allowing the patient to be more vigorous with oral hygiene. The firmer keratinized tissue may therefore protect the implants and improve their prognosis by decreasing

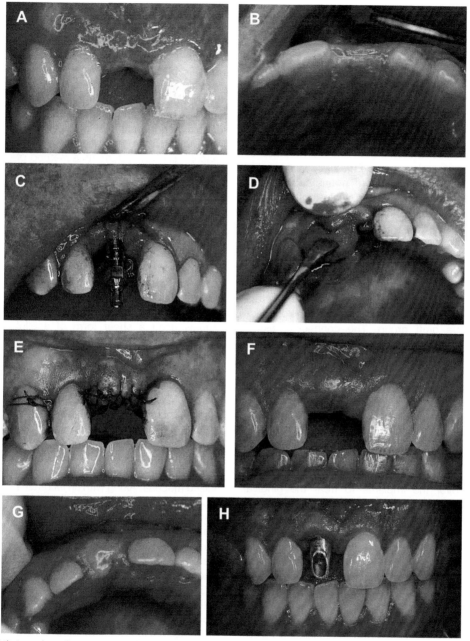

Fig. 4. (*A*) An edentulous space with loss in vertical dimension. (*B*) Occlusal view indicating the loss in bucco-lingual dimensions. This is a Siebert class III ridge deformity. (*C*) The ridge was expanded and the implant placed. (*D*) A rotated split palatal graft was prepared and rolled over the implant site. (*E*) Suturing of the site. (*F*) Healing after 6 months. (*G*) The occlusal view of the healing after 6 months. (*H*) The gingival zenith at time of abutment placement.

potential discomfort and inflammation that could occur from vigorous oral hygiene at a mucosal implant interface.

In fully edentulous implant reconstructions, vestibuloplasty and free gingival tissue grafting techniques have been used to obtain attached keratinized tissue in the anterior edentulous mandible before implant placement in an effort to improve the long-term prognosis.[92] To a lesser extent, free gingival grafts have been used in immediate implant placement. A graft is obtained with a biopsy punch from the palate, and then it is used to cover the exposed surface of the implant without repositioning the mucoperiosteal flap.

Free Connective Grafts

The use of subepithelial connective tissue grafts around dental implants was a natural extension from their use to cover exposed root surfaces with greater predictability and superior clinical gingival color match compared with free gingival grafts.[93] Connective tissue grafts have been used as a soft-tissue barrier to close over an immediate postextraction implant as a soft-tissue extension over a barrier membrane or in place of the barrier membrane (see **Fig. 2**).[94,95]

Immediate implant placement and subepithelial connective tissue grafts for single-tooth restoration versus immediate implant alone were studied for preservation of keratinized mucosa amount and bone tissue, optimal peri-implant marginal sealing, and esthetic outcomes.[95] The 9-year cumulative survival rate was 100% for test and control groups. Comparative statistical analysis of soft- and hard-tissue peri-implant parameters showed a more favorable outcome for the connective tissue graft group. The connective tissue group showed good results in terms of esthetic parameters, which estimated the keratinized mucosa width, the alignment of crown emergence profile, and the patient's satisfaction.

Covani and colleagues[96] extracted teeth and placed implants after periodontal treatment on teeth deemed to have a poor prognosis. The teeth were extracted and implants were placed without reflection of a mucoperiosteal flap. Immediately after implantation, a connective tissue graft was placed over the implants to treat the gingival recession. The investigators considered the surgical approach used in this study to be a viable treatment option in cases with nonsalvageable teeth showing gingival recession and the absence of attached gingiva.

In a prospective case series to evaluate the healing outcome of soft-tissue dehiscence coverage at implant sites, 10 patients with 1 mucosal recession defect at an implant site and a contralateral unrestored clinical crown without recession were recruited.[97] The soft-tissue recessions were surgically covered using a coronally advanced flap in combination with a free connective tissue graft. The implant sites revealed a 66% coverage of the dehiscence and clinically significant improvement following coronal mucosal displacement in combination with connective tissue grafting; however, complete implant soft-tissue dehiscence coverage could not be achieved in all sites.

Even in cases without recession pre-extraction, once the gingival fibers inserting into the tooth are severed there is a tendency for gingival collapse and apical migration of the gingival margin. This apical migration on the implant surface potentially leads to an esthetic compromise (**Fig. 5**). Immediate implant placement and provisionalization has been considered a preservative procedure when replacing failing teeth, especially in the esthetic zone. Nevertheless, an average facial gingival tissue recession of 1 mm is still common after 1 year of function. Facial gingival recession of thin periodontal biotype seems to be more pronounced than that of thick biotype. For that reason, gingival grafting as a method of changing the gingival phenotype of natural teeth and implants with subepithelial connective tissue graft has been advocated. The resulting tissues seem to be more resistant to recession.[98]

Soft-tissue Allografts

Initial reports examined the clinical efficacy of acellular dermal matrix allograft to achieve increased peri-implant keratinized mucosa around[99–108] implants. These proof-of-concept studies used a sheet form of acellular dermal matrix allograft to increase the attached keratinized mucosa. Park[99] found a statistical difference in pocket depth and modified plaque index at 6 months compared with the baseline measurements. The width of peri-implant keratinized mucosa increased from a mean of 0.8 ± 0.6 mm to 2.2 ± 0.6 mm at 6 months. Based on these findings, there is potential that an acellular dermal matrix allograft could be applied as a grafting material to increase the width of peri-implant keratinized mucosa. Along with an increase in attached tissue, there are some benefits for oral hygiene. Further long-term randomized controlled trials are necessary to establish the use of acellular dermal allografts compared with free gingival grafts or subepithelial connective tissue grafts for long-term benefits to patients.

Geurs and colleagues[100] investigated the application of micronized acellular dermal graft for the reconstruction of papillae around teeth. The micronized allograft technique showed promise for the repair of interproximal areas of tissue loss.

Buccal augmentation with acellular dermal grafting has been used to thicken the peri-implant mucosa to mask the shine-through of a gray cast from an implant abutment or collar in which the host tissue biotype is thin (**Fig. 6**). This technique in preliminary reports has been effective in improving the esthetics along with the increase in tissue thickness. In addition, facial acellular dermal grafts have been used in combination with particulate bone grafts to augment tissue on the facial surface of implants.[101] Although there is limited evidence of regeneration of bone around these

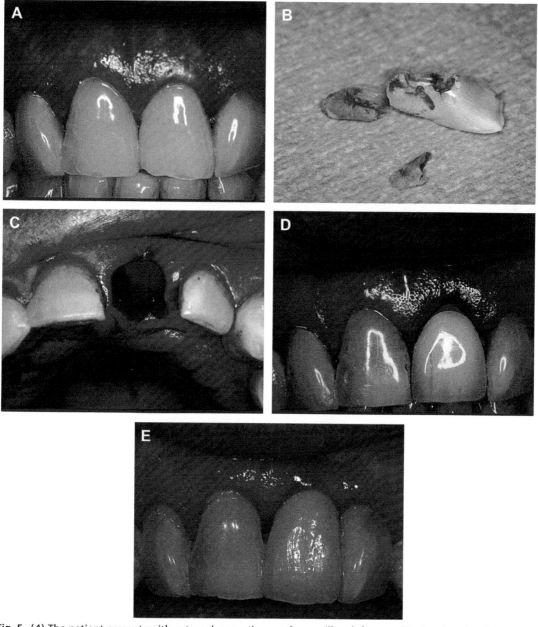

Fig. 5. (*A*) The patient presents with external resorption on the maxillary left central incisor (tooth #9), with the gingival margin located slightly more incisal than the adjacent central incisor (tooth #8). (*B*) The resorption was located on the palatal surface of the tooth and, after extraction with a periotome technique, the facial plate of bone was intact. (*C*) An occlusal view indicating limited or no loss of adjacent soft-tissue support. (*D*) Insertion of a provisional restoration made at the same clinical crown height of the natural tooth indicating the immediate loss of soft-tissue support without the gingival fiber support provided by the extracted tooth. (*E*) Final implant-supported crown with a compromised esthetic result due to the loss of soft vertical margin height after extraction.

augmentation sites, there seems to be a predictable improvement in the esthetics in anterior areas. Acellular dermal grafting has also been used as a form of barrier membrane for guided tissue regeneration. Although the primary indication for the soft-tissue allograft in these applications is containment of the graft to allow for organization of the blood clot, the dermal allograft may also serve to augment the thickness of the mucosa in the area of the implant.[102,103]

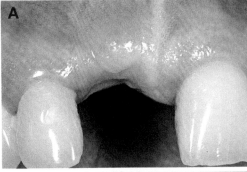

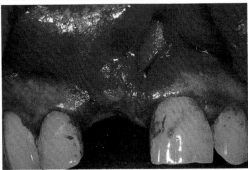

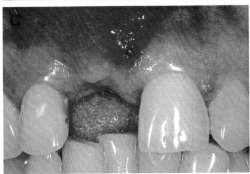

Fig. 6. (A) Patient with a gray cast or shine-through due to the collar of the implant under relatively thin mucosa. (B) Tunneling of an acellular dermal graft over the implant collar through a single vertical incision in the vestibule to limit interruption of blood supply to the region. (C) The initial healing illustrating masking of the implant collar color by thickening the over mucosa.

Combination Hard- and Soft-tissue Grafting

The combination of bone grafting and soft-tissue augmentation has been used for site preparation. The technique used may incorporate a particulate bone graft, growth factors, and barrier membrane along with a pedicle or free connective tissue graft to simultaneously augment the hard and soft tissue. In patients with the loss of the facial plate and requiring extraction of anterior teeth, combined approaches may be advantageous. Although there is an increasing level of complexity

when multiple techniques and materials are combined into a single wound-healing procedure, there is clinical evidence of the potential effectiveness of this technique in delayed- and immediate-implant cases.

LIMITING ESTHETIC PROBLEMS AROUND IMPLANTS
Buccal Augmentation

One of the most difficult esthetic soft-tissue situations is the extraction of a single tooth or multiple anterior teeth and replacement with implants. The loss of the facial plate complicates the situation and further compromises the esthetics. Severing interdental fibers attached to the tooth almost universally leads to some loss of soft-tissue height and subsequent recession of the tissue. In a retrospective study, the soft-tissue and esthetic outcomes at single-tooth immediate implants placed without flap elevation in maxillary central and lateral incisor sites was evaluated. Chen and colleagues[104] recorded the mucosal level of 85 consecutive patients. In this study, the change in mucosal level was expressed as a percentage of the length of the reference central incisor. Significant recession of the mesial papilla ($-6.2\% \pm 6.8\%$), distal papilla ($-7.4\% \pm 7.5\%$), and facial mucosa ($-4.6\% \pm 6.6\%$) between surgical placement and 1 year was observed. Recession was significantly greater for implants placed facially within the extraction socket compared with those placed lingually. Sites with gingival margins initially coronal achieved mucosal levels close to the line of symmetry with the contralateral tooth. Sites initially level or apical failed to reach the line of symmetry and remained receded. For sites with initially level gingival margins, recession greater than 10% occurred at 6 of 25 thin-biotype sites compared with 2 of 19 thick-biotype sites.

This study shows that immediate implant placement, even without elevation of surgical flaps, was associated with recession of the marginal mucosa. This finding underscores the need to consider the placement of the implant away from the facial surface and the assessment of the biotype during implant treatment planning. In addition, if esthetics are a major treatment consideration, augmentation of the soft tissue incisal to the adjacent teeth may limit the potential for recession during restoration.

Papilla Grafting

Implant papilla loss is often the result of limitations imposed by the quantity of the supporting bone, periodontal bone loss on adjacent teeth, and bone volume and direct effect on the soft-tissue biotype in the region. Because of these limitations, there are frequent situations in which implants are placed in areas of minimal interproximal soft tissue that can result in dark triangles between crowns and crown margins that become supragingival. Both of these can lead to a poor esthetic outcome that is often disappointing for the patient and the practitioner. Several procedures have been described to improve the interproximal papillae contour around implants. Grunder[105] described the inlay graft technique to create papillae between teeth. Azzi and colleagues[106] outlined a technique of tunneling/pouching and the use of submerged connective tissue grafts. This technique allows for the thickening of the existing gingiva but is also potentially useful for reconstructing interdental papillae around implant-supported restorations. Reddy[107] described a tunneling connective tissue grafting technique with access through a vertical incision in the vestibule that allowed for vertical augmentation of the papillae with minimal interruption to the blood supply in the region. Although these techniques collectively have been successful in re-establishing papillae at implant sites, the papillary soft-tissue grafting is much less complicated to achieve when attempted before the restoration of the implant with a crown.

Provisional Restorations

The selection of the type of provisional restoration can significantly influence esthetics during the period of implant integration and soft-tissue healing.[108] A restoration that preserves or helps to regenerate interdental papillae will enhance the final esthetic result of the soft tissue (**Fig. 7**). The importance of establishing proper contours in the provisional restoration should be part of the treatment plan for any esthetic implant case. A provisional restoration was used immediately after extraction to preserve the interdental papillae. Whenever possible, a fixed restoration should be considered as a good alternative to removable provisional restorations. The contour of the soft tissue is largely dictated by the crown contact points and emergence profile during healing.

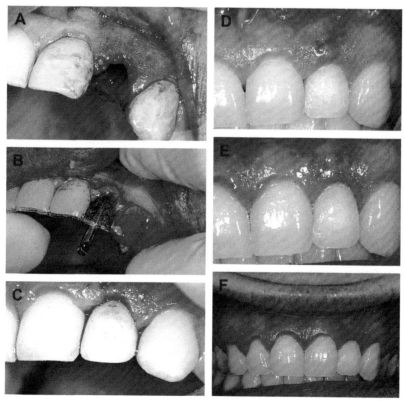

Fig. 7. (*A*) Atraumatic extraction of a fractured tooth. (*B*) Immediate implant placement with a surgical guide. (*C*) Provisional restoration to establish soft-tissue contour and esthetics without functional loading. (*D*) Initial healing response of the soft tissue after 1 week. (*E*) Healing response to provisional soft-tissue support after 1 month. (*F*) Two months after immediate implant placement and establishment of gingival contours relative to anterior teeth.

All of these aspects of soft-tissue healing, implant design, and maintenance of soft tissue around dental implants need to be considered before implant placement. In treatment planning, the proper sequence of site development of the hard and soft tissue needs to be made with the biology of the final restoration in mind.

REFERENCES

1. Berglundh T, Lindhe J, Ericsson I, et al. The soft tissue barrier at implants and teeth. Clin Oral Implants Res 1991;2(2):81–90.
2. Buser D, Weber H, Donath K, et al. Soft tissue reactions to non-submerged unloaded titanium implants in beagle dogs. J Periodontol 1992;63(3):225–35.
3. Berglundh T, Abrahamsson I, Welander M, et al. Morphogenesis of the peri-implant mucosa: an experimental study in dogs. Clin Oral Implants Res 2007;18(1):1–8.
4. Gould T, Westbury L, Brunette D. Ultrastructural study of the attachment of human gingiva to titanium in vivo. J Prosthet Dent 1984;52(3):418–20.
5. Steflik D, Corpe R, Young T, et al. The biologic tissue responses to uncoated and coated implanted biomaterials. Adv Dent Res 1999;13:27–33.
6. Listgarten M. Soft and hard tissue response to endosseous dental implants. Anat Rec 1996;245(2):410–25.
7. Chehroudi B, Gould T, Brunette D. The role of connective tissue in inhibiting epithelial downgrowth on titanium-coated percutaneous implants. J Biomed Mater Res 1992;26(4):493–515.
8. Nevins M, Nevins M, Camelo M, et al. Human histologic evidence of a connective tissue attachment to a dental implant. Int J Periodontics Restorative Dent 2008;28(2):111–21.
9. Abrahamsson I, Zitzmann N, Berglundh T, et al. The mucosal attachment to titanium implants with different surface characteristics: an experimental study in dogs. J Clin Periodontol 2002; 29(5):448–55.
10. Berglundh T, Lindhe J. Dimension of the periimplant mucosa. Biological width revisited. J Clin Periodontol 1996;23(10):971–3.
11. Stern I. Current concepts of the dentogingival junction: the epithelial and connective tissue attachments to the tooth. J Periodontol 1981; 52(9):465–76.
12. Ericsson I, Lindhe J. Probing depth at implants and teeth. An experimental study in the dog. J Clin Periodontol 1993;20(9):623–7.
13. Broggini N, McManus L, Hermann J, et al. Peri-implant inflammation defined by the implant-abutment interface. J Dent Res 2006;85(5):473–8.
14. Teté S, Mastrangelo F, Bianchi A, et al. Collagen fiber orientation around machined titanium and zirconia dental implant necks: an animal study. Int J Oral Maxillofac Implants 2009;24(1):52–8.
15. Traini T, Degidi M, Caputi S, et al. Collagen fiber orientation in human peri-implant bone around immediately loaded and unloaded titanium dental implants. J Periodontol 2005;76(1):83–9.
16. Traini T, Pecora G, Iezzi G, et al. Preferred collagen fiber orientation human peri-implant bone after a short- and long-term loading period: a case report. J Oral Implantol 2006;32(4):177–81.
17. Schwarz F, Ferrari D, Herten M, et al. Effects of surface hydrophilicity and microtopography on early stages of soft and hard tissue integration at non-submerged titanium implants: an immunohistochemical study in dogs. J Periodontol 2007; 78(11):2171–84.
18. Moon I, Berglundh T, Abrahamsson I, et al. The barrier between the keratinized mucosa and the dental implant. An experimental study in the dog. J Clin Periodontol 1999;26(10):658–63.
19. Abrahamsson I, Berglundh T, Glantz P, et al. The mucosal attachment at different abutments. An experimental study in dogs. J Clin Periodontol 1998;25(9):721–7.
20. Romanos G, Schröter-Kermani C, Weingart D, et al. Health human periodontal versus peri-implant gingival tissues: an immunohistochemical differentiation of the extracellular matrix. Int J Oral Maxillofac Implants 2009;10(6):750–8.
21. Davies J. Mechanisms of endosseous integration. Int J Prosthodont 1998;11(5):391–401.
22. Davies J. Understanding peri-implant endosseous healing. J Dent Educ 2003;67(8):932–49.
23. Araújo M, Lindhe J. Dimensional ridge alterations following tooth extraction. An experimental study in the dog. J Clin Periodontol 2005;32(2):212–8.
24. Kim B, Kim Y, Yun P, et al. Evaluation of peri-implant tissue response according to the presence of keratinized mucosa. Oral Surg Oral Med Oral Pathol Oral Radiol Endod 2009;107(3):e24–8.
25. Abrahamsson I, Berglundh T, Lindhe J. The mucosal barrier following abutment dis/reconnection. An experimental study in dogs. J Clin Periodontol 1997;24(8):568–72.
26. Linkevicius T, Apse P, Grybauskas S, et al. The influence of soft tissue thickness on crestal bone changes around implants: a 1-year prospective controlled clinical trial. Int J Oral Maxillofac Implants 2009;24(4):712–9.
27. Cairo F, Pagliaro U, Nieri M. Soft tissue management at implant sites. J Clin Periodontol 2008; 35(Suppl 8):163–7.
28. Bouri AJ, Bissada N, Al-Zahrani M, et al. Width of keratinized gingiva and the health status of the supporting tissues around dental implants. Int J Oral Maxillofac Implants 2008;23(2):323–6.

29. Klinge B, Flemmig T. Tissue augmentation and esthetics (Working Group 3). Clin Oral Implants Res 2009;20(Suppl 4):166–70.

30. Kois J. Predictable single-tooth peri-implant esthetics: five diagnostic keys. Compend Contin Educ Dent 2004;25(11):895–6 898, 900 passim [quiz: 906–7].

31. Jung R, Holderegger C, Sailer I, et al. The effect of all-ceramic and porcelain-fused-to-metal restorations on marginal peri-implant soft tissue color: a randomized controlled clinical trial. Int J Periodontics Restorative Dent 2008;28(4):357–65.

32. Gargiulo AW, Wentz FM, Orban B. Dimensions and relations of the dentogingival junction in humans. J Periodontol 1961;32:261–7.

33. Perez J, Smukler H, Nunn M. Clinical evaluation of the supraosseous gingivae before and after crown lengthening. J Periodontol 2007;78(6):1023–30.

34. Barboza E, MonteAlto R, Ferreira V, et al. Supracrestal gingival tissue measurements in healthy human periodontium. Int J Periodontics Restorative Dent 2008;28(1):55–61.

35. Vacek J, Gher M, Assad D, et al. The dimensions of the human dentogingival junction. Int J Periodontics Restorative Dent 1994;14(2):154–65.

36. Maynard JJ, Wilson R. Physiologic dimensions of the periodontium significant to the restorative dentist. J Periodontol 1979;50(4):170–4.

37. Abrahamsson I, Berglundh T, Moon I, et al. Peri-implant tissues at submerged and non-submerged titanium implants. J Clin Periodontol 1999;26(9):600–7.

38. Hermann J, Buser D, Schenk R, et al. Biologic width around titanium implants. A physiologically formed and stable dimension over time. Clin Oral Implants Res 2000;11(1):1–11.

39. Hermann J, Buser D, Schenk R, et al. Biologic width around one- and two-piece titanium implants. Clin Oral Implants Res 2001;12(6):559–71.

40. Bakaeen L, Quinlan P, Schoolfield J, et al. The biologic width around titanium implants: histometric analysis of the implantogingival junction around immediately and early loaded implants. Int J Periodontics Restorative Dent 2009;29(3):297–305.

41. Buser D, Mericske-Stern R, Bernard J, et al. Long-term evaluation of non-submerged ITI implants. Part 1: 8-year life table analysis of a prospective multi-center study with 2359 implants. Clin Oral Implants Res 1997;8(3):161–72.

42. Hermann J, Cochran D, Nummikoski P, et al. Crestal bone changes around titanium implants. A radiographic evaluation of unloaded nonsubmerged and submerged implants in the canine mandible. J Periodontol 1997;68(11):1117–30.

43. Quirynen M, van Steenberghe D. Bacterial colonization of the internal part of two-stage implants. An in vivo study. Clin Oral Implants Res 1993; 4(3):158–61.

44. Tarnow D, Cho S, Wallace S. The effect of inter-implant distance on the height of inter-implant bone crest. J Periodontol 2000;71(4):546–9.

45. Hermann J, Schoolfield J, Schenk R, et al. Influence of the size of the microgap on crestal bone changes around titanium implants. A histometric evaluation of unloaded non-submerged implants in the canine mandible. J Periodontol 2001; 72(10):1372–83.

46. Piattelli A, Vrespa G, Petrone G, et al. Role of the microgap between implant and abutment: a retrospective histologic evaluation in monkeys. J Periodontol 2003;74(3):346–52.

47. Todescan F, Pustiglioni F, Imbronito A, et al. Influence of the microgap in the peri-implant hard and soft tissues: a histomorphometric study in dogs. Int J Oral Maxillofac Implants 2002; 17(4):467–72.

48. Van Assche N, Collaert B, Coucke W, et al. Correlation between early perforation of cover screws and marginal bone loss: a retrospective study. J Clin Periodontol 2008;35(1):76–9.

49. Tal H. Spontaneous early exposure of submerged implants: I. Classification and clinical observations. J Periodontol 1999;70(2):213–9.

50. Tal H, Artzi Z, Moses O, et al. Spontaneous early exposure of submerged endosseous implants resulting in crestal bone loss: a clinical evaluation between stage I and stage II surgery. Int J Oral Maxillofac Implants 2001;16(4):514–21.

51. Jeong S, Choi B, Li J, et al. The effect of thick mucosa on peri-implant tissues: an experimental study in dogs. J Periodontol 2008;79(11): 2151–5.

52. Cosyn J, Sabzevar M, De Wilde P, et al. Two-piece implants with turned versus microtextured collars. J Periodontol 2007;78(9):1657–63.

53. Subramani K, Jung R, Molenberg A, et al. Biofilm on dental implants: a review of the literature. Int J Oral Maxillofac Implants 2009;24(4):616–26.

54. Trammell K, Geurs N, O'Neal SJ, et al. A prospective, randomized, controlled comparison of platform-switched and matched-abutment implants in short-span partial denture situations. Int J Periodontics Restorative Dent 2009;29:599–605.

55. López-Marí L, Calvo-Guirado J, Martín-Castellote B, et al. Implant platform switching concept: an updated review. Med Oral Patol Oral Cir Bucal 2009;14(9):e450–4.

56. Hürzeler M, Fickl S, Zuhr O, et al. Peri-implant bone level around implants with platform-switched abutments: preliminary data from a prospective study. J Oral Maxillofac Surg 2007;65(7 Suppl 1):33–9.

57. Weiner S, Simon J, Ehrenberg D, et al. The effects of laser microtextured collars upon crestal bone levels of dental implants. Implant Dent 2008; 17(2):217–28.

58. Pecora G, Ceccarelli R, Bonelli M, et al. Clinical evaluation of laser microtexturing for soft tissue and bone attachment to dental implants. Implant Dent 2009;18(1):57–66.

59. Tarnow D, Magner A, Fletcher P. The effect of the distance from the contact point to the crest of bone on the presence or absence of the interproximal dental papilla. J Periodontol 1992;63(12):995–6.

60. Choquet V, Hermans M, Adriaenssens P, et al. Clinical and radiographic evaluation of the papilla level adjacent to single-tooth dental implants. A retrospective study in the maxillary anterior region. J Periodontol 2001;72(10):1364–71.

61. Jemt T. Regeneration of gingival papillae after single-implant treatment. Int J Periodontics Restorative Dent 1997;17(4):326–33.

62. Kourkouta S, Dedi K, Paquette D, et al. Interproximal tissue dimensions in relation to adjacent implants in the anterior maxilla: clinical observations and patient aesthetic evaluation. Clin Oral Implants Res 2009;20(12):1375–85.

63. Tarnow D, Elian N, Fletcher P, et al. Vertical distance from the crest of bone to the height of the interproximal papilla between adjacent implants. J Periodontol 2003;74(12):1785–8.

64. Reddy M, O'Neal S, Haigh S, et al. Initial clinical efficacy of 3-mm implants immediately placed into function in conditions of limited spacing. Int J Oral Maxillofac Implants 2008;23(2):281–8.

65. Weber HP, Buser D, Belser UC. Examination of the candidate for implant therapy. In: Lang NP, Lindhe J, editors. Clinical periodontology and implant dentistry, vol. 1. 5th edition. Ames (IA): Blackwell Publishing; 2009. p. 587–97.

66. Warrer K, Buser D, Lang N, et al. Plaque-induced peri-implantitis in the presence or absence of keratinized mucosa. An experimental study in monkeys. Clin Oral Implants Res 1995;6(3):131–8.

67. Schrott A, Jimenez M, Hwang J, et al. Five-year evaluation of the influence of keratinized mucosa on peri-implant soft-tissue health and stability around implants supporting full-arch mandibular fixed prostheses. Clin Oral Implants Res 2009;20(10):1170–7.

68. Wennström J, Bengazi F, Lekholm U. The influence of the masticatory mucosa on the peri-implant soft tissue condition. Clin Oral Implants Res 1994;5(1):1–8.

69. Cooper L. Objective criteria: guiding and evaluating dental implant esthetics. J Esthet Restor Dent 2008;20(3):195–205.

70. Kopp FR, Belser U. Esthetic checklist for the fixed prosthesis. In: Sharer P, Kopp FR, Rinn LA, editors. Esthetic guidelines for restorative dentistry. Chicago (IL): Quintessence Publishing Co; 1982. p. 187–92.

71. Wilson D. Ridge mapping for determination of alveolar ridge width. Int J Oral Maxillofac Implants 1989;4(1):41–3.

72. Olsson M, Lindhe J. Periodontal characteristics in individuals with varying form of the upper central incisors. J Clin Periodontol 1991;18(1):78–82.

73. Weisgold A. Contours of the full crown restoration. Alpha Omegan 1977;70(3):77–89.

74. Olsson M, Lindhe J, Marinello C. On the relationship between crown form and clinical features of the gingiva in adolescents. J Clin Periodontol 1993;20(8):570–7.

75. Becker W, Ochsenbein C, Tibbetts L, et al. Alveolar bone anatomic profiles as measured from dry skulls. Clinical ramifications. J Clin Periodontol 1997;24(10):727–31.

76. Seibert JS. Reconstruction of deformed, partially edentulous ridges, using full thickness onlay grafts. I. Technique and wound healing. Compend Contin Educ Dent 1983;4:437–53.

77. Palacci P, Nowzari H. Soft tissue enhancement around dental implants. Periodontol 2000 2008; 47:113–32.

78. Priest G. The esthetic challenge of adjacent implants. J Oral Maxillofac Surg 2007;65(7 Suppl 1):2–12.

79. Grunder U, Gracis S, Capelli M. Influence of the 3-D bone-to-implant relationship on esthetics. Int J Periodontics Restorative Dent 2005;25(2):113–9.

80. Kan J, Rungcharassaeng K. Interimplant papilla preservation in the esthetic zone: a report of six consecutive cases. Int J Periodontics Restorative Dent 2003;23(3):249–59.

81. Magne P, Belser U. Bonded porcelain restorations in the anterior dentition. A biomimetic approach. Carol Stream (IL): Quintessence; 2002.

82. Rufenacht CR. Principles of esthetic integration. Chicago (IL): Quintessence Publishing; 2000.

83. Esposito M, Ekestubbe A, Gröndahl K. Radiological evaluation of marginal bone loss at tooth surfaces facing single Brånemark implants. Clin Oral Implants Res 1993;4(3):151–7.

84. Gasparini D. Double-fold connective tissue pedicle graft: a novel approach for ridge augmentation. Int J Periodontics Restorative Dent 2004;24(3):280–7.

85. Adell R, Eriksson B, Lekholm U, et al. Long-term follow-up study of osseointegrated implants in the treatment of totally edentulous jaws. Int J Oral Maxillofac Implants 1990;5(4):347–59.

86. Becker W, Becker B. Guided tissue regeneration for implants placed into extraction sockets and for implant dehiscences: surgical techniques and case report. Int J Periodontics Restorative Dent 1990;10(5):376–91.

87. Goldstein M, Boyan B, Schwartz Z. The palatal advanced flap: a pedicle flap for primary coverage of immediately placed implants. Clin Oral Implants Res 2002;13(6):644–50.

88. Nemcovsky C, Artzi Z, Moses O. Rotated split palatal flap for soft tissue primary coverage

over extraction sites with immediate implant placement. Description of the surgical procedure and clinical results. J Periodontol 1999;70 (8):926–34.

89. Nemcovsky C, Artzi Z, Moses O. Rotated palatal flap in immediate implant procedures. Clinical evaluation of 26 consecutive cases. Clin Oral Implants Res 2000;11(1):83–90.

90. Khoury F, Happe A. The palatal subepithelial connective tissue flap method for soft tissue management to cover maxillary defects: a clinical report. Int J Oral Maxillofac Implants 2000;15(3): 415–8.

91. Simons A, Darany D, Giordano J. The use of free gingival grafts in the treatment of peri-implant soft tissue complications: clinical report. Implant Dent 1993;2(1):27–30.

92. Hoelscher D, Simons A. The rationale for soft-tissue grafting and vestibuloplasty in association with endosseous implants: a literature review. J Oral Implantol 1994;20(4):282–91.

93. Langer B, Calagna L. The subepithelial connective tissue graft. J Prosthet Dent 1980;44(4):363–7.

94. Edel A. The use of a connective tissue graft for closure over an immediate implant covered with occlusive membrane. Clin Oral Implants Res 1995;6(1):60–5.

95. Bianchi A, Sanfilippo F. Single-tooth replacement by immediate implant and connective tissue graft: a 1-9-year clinical evaluation. Clin Oral Implants Res 2004;15(3):269–77.

96. Covani U, Marconcini S, Galassini G, et al. Connective tissue graft used as a biologic barrier to cover an immediate implant. J Periodontol 2007;78(8): 1644–9.

97. Burkhardt R, Joss A, Lang N. Soft tissue dehiscence coverage around endosseous implants: a prospective cohort study. Clin Oral Implants Res 2008;19(5):451–7.

98. Kan J, Rungcharassaeng K, Lozada J. Bilaminar subepithelial connective tissue grafts for immediate implant placement and provisionalization in the esthetic zone. J Calif Dent Assoc 2005; 33(11):865–71.

99. Park J. Increasing the width of keratinized mucosa around endosseous implant using acellular dermal matrix allograft. Implant Dent 2006;15(3):275–81.

100. Geurs N, Romanos A, Vassilopoulos P, et al. Efficacy of micronized acellular dermal graft for use in interproximal papillae regeneration. Int J Periodontics Restorative Dent, in press.

101. Park S, Wang H. Management of localized buccal dehiscence defect with allografts and acellular dermal matrix. Int J Periodontics Restorative Dent 2006;26(6):589–95.

102. El Helow K, El Askary AS. Regenerative barriers in immediate implant placement: a literature review. Implant Dent 2008;17(3):360–71.

103. Park S, Lee K, Oh T, et al. Effect of absorbable membranes on sandwich bone augmentation. Clin Oral Implants Res 2008;19(1):32–41.

104. Chen S, Darby I, Reynolds E, et al. Immediate implant placement postextraction without flap elevation. J Periodontol 2009;80(1):163–72.

105. Grunder U. The inlay-graft technique to create papillae between implants. J Esthet Dent 1997; 9(4):165–8.

106. Azzi R, Etienne D, Takei H, et al. Surgical thickening of the existing gingiva and reconstruction of interdental papillae around implant-supported restorations. Int J Periodontics Restorative Dent 2002;22(1):71–7.

107. Reddy M. Achieving gingival esthetics. J Am Dent Assoc 2003;134(3):295–304 [quiz: 337–8].

108. Sachdeva K, Kula K, Hains F. Provisional restoration to preserve interdental papillae in the esthetic zone: a case report. J Indiana Dent Assoc 2009; 88(1):31–5.

Dental Implants After Reconstruction with Free Tissue Transfer

Jon D. Holmes, DMD, MD[a,b,*],
Ruth Aponte-Wesson, DDS, MS[c]

KEYWORDS

- Dental implants • Implants • Free flaps
- Free tissue transfer • Oral cavity reconstruction

Most contemporary techniques for reconstructing composite defects of the oral cavity resulting from oncologic resections, or avulsive traumatic injuries, typically involve some type of free tissue transfer via microvascular techniques. The ability to transfer composite tissue flaps or free flaps from distant sites to the head and neck by microvascular techniques revolutionized oral cavity reconstruction. Free tissue transfer allows immediate, 1-step reconstruction of complex defects that previously required multistaged efforts with less-than-ideal results and has demonstrated an increased success in reconstruction of large defects compared with nonvascularized grafting techniques.[1,2] Although a variety of flaps that provide excellent esthetic and functional reconstructions are available, dental rehabilitation remains challenging. For a dental prosthesis to be effective, one should remember the basic principles that make it successful, including retention, stability, and support. When natural anatomy has been altered due to ablative surgical procedures, trauma, or a congenital abnormality, some of these basic principles for prosthesis success are compromised. To reestablish the loss of contours and some of the basic principles, the use of sophisticated reconstructive methods and adjunct osseointegrated implants has been advocated. To have acceptable results, extensive planning and understanding should exist among all team members. The degree of success is in direct relationship to the location and extent of the mandibular resection, amount of adjacent soft tissue removed in the surgical procedure, and the presence or absence of natural teeth.[3]

The imported tissue lacks many of the characteristics of the native tissue it is replacing and rarely recapitulates the anatomy perfectly (**Fig. 1**). In addition, patients who have undergone reconstruction often suffer from significant trismus secondary to scarring and radiation fibrosis. The maximum size of the opening, not infrequently less than 20 mm, makes conventional prosthetic techniques inadequate (**Fig. 2**).

For these reasons, traditional dental restorative techniques are typically insufficient, and dental implants are required to provide stabilization and retention of prostheses. Similarly, the flaps themselves often do not provide the ideal site for implant placement. Reports on the success of endosseous implants placed in conjunction with free flaps often focus solely on the successful integration of the fixture while paying less attention to the prosthetic outcome. The primary impediments to implant placement and long-term maintenance in flaps imported as microvascular transfers are the characteristics of the soft and hard tissues. This article describes site development and prosthetic

---

[a] Private practice, Oral and Facial Surgery of Alabama, 1500, 19th Street South, Birmingham, AL 35205, USA
[b] Department of Oral and Maxillofacial Surgery, University of Alabama at Birmingham, 1919 7th Avenue South, Birmingham, AL 35294, USA
[c] Department of Prosthodontics, School of Dentistry Building, University of Alabama at Birmingham, 1919 7th Avenue South, Birmingham, AL 35294, USA
* Corresponding author. Private practice, Oral and Facial Surgery of Alabama, 1500, 19th Street South, Birmingham, AL 35205.
E-mail address: j-holmes@mindspring.com

Oral Maxillofacial Surg Clin N Am 22 (2010) 407–418
doi:10.1016/j.coms.2010.04.002

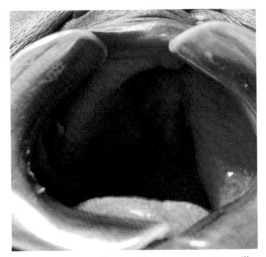

Fig. 1. Bulky rectus flap used to reconstruct maxillectomy defect provides closure of defect but precludes any prosthetic rehabilitation.

techniques that can be applied in an attempt to overcome some of these shortcomings of free flap reconstructions for oral cavity defects.

RADIATION AND OSSEOINTEGRATION

Before discussing specific surgical and prosthetic maneuvers that can be performed to develop the physical site for implant placement and maintenance, mention should be made of the potential role of hyperbaric oxygen (HBO) therapy in the site preparation for patients who have received radiation therapy. Although it is beyond the scope of this article to completely review the controversy surrounding the role of HBO therapy, readers should be aware of the questions surrounding its use. More extensive reviews are available.[4,5]

Frequently, oncologic patients who require free tissue transfer for reconstruction also qualify for multimodality therapy, including radiation and/or chemotherapy. Radiation therapy may have been administered before, or after, the resection and

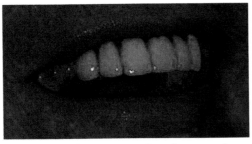

Fig. 2. Patient after reconstruction of segmental mandibulectomy defect followed by radiation therapy presenting with significant scarring and fibrosis and a maximum interincisal opening of less than 10 mm.

reconstruction. Radiation therapy has known consequences on the response of soft tissue and bone to surgical wounding. In addition, long-term effects on the mucosa and salivary function affect the maintenance of natural dentition as well as integrated implants. Based primarily on the work of Marx and colleagues,[6–8] prophylactic HBO therapy has been recommended before extraction of teeth for the prevention of osteoradionecrosis (ORN) and is also promoted for the treatment. The role of HBO in the treatment of established ORN has come under increased scrutiny after a double-blind placebo-controlled trial, which was halted early because the hyperbaric treatment arm was fairing worse than the placebo treatment arm.[9] Similar findings were demonstrated by Gal and colleagues,[10] who found worse outcomes in patients undergoing surgical treatment for established ORN, including resection and free tissue reconstruction, than those patients who received HBO therapy. Similarly, the role of prophylactic HBO therapy in preventing ORN is increasingly being questioned, and still more controversial is the role of HBO in the irradiated patient who is to undergo implant placement.

After the introduction of the concept of osseointegration and its promotion as a potential technique for dental rehabilitation of the oncologic patient, questions were raised regarding the need for prophylactic HBO therapy. Several investigators have attempted to answer the question of whether or not a protocol incorporating HBO administration before and after dental implant placement (typically 20 dives and 10 dives following, with each dive consisting of 90 minutes at 2.4 atm) increases the chances of successful integration and whether or not it aids in long-term maintenance. Initially, Marx's work on a prophylactic protocol of HBO before dental extractions in irradiated patients was extrapolated to irradiated patients scheduled for implant placement. Granstrom's[11] work concluded that administering HBO increased the success rate of integration in all sites studied, and hence it should be administered. The study, however, included a heterogeneous population with a significant number of extraoral fixtures and a minority of intraoral implants. Other investigators including Eckert and colleagues[12] who reported a 99% implant survival rate for 89 implants placed in irradiated mandibles without HBO therapy have argued against routinely administering HBO before implant placement. Overall, the reported rate of ORN has been less than 5% in patients who did not receive HBO therapy before implant placement in oral sites.[13] Similarly, Schoen and colleagues[14] demonstrated no difference in their prospective study of patients undergoing placement of dental implants in the anterior mandible. Patients were randomized into a group receiving antibiotic prophylaxis and another group receiving antibiotics and pre- and postoperative HBO therapy. The rate of nonosseointegration was higher in the HBO group (85.2%) than the non-HBO group (93.9%), and the only case of ORN in the study developed in a patient in the HBO group. Importantly, this study addressed only implants placed in native mandibular bone. Many of the ongoing questions surrounding the use of prophylactic HBO therapy before implant placement are illustrated by Granstrom[15] and Donoff[16] taking opposing views. However, neither specifically addressed the issue of implants placed in irradiated areas reconstructed with free tissue transfer. Aside from adding treatment time, HBO therapy is expensive. In many countries, including the United States, dental implant placement is considered elective by insurance carriers and costs are borne solely by the patient, making prophylactic HBO therapy cost-prohibitive in many cases. A review by Esposito and colleagues[17] failed to demonstrate benefit of HBO therapy in irradiated patients undergoing placement of dental implants. In addition to questions of costs and benefits, from a practical standpoint HBO therapy may not be available in all areas.

Cuesta-Gil and colleagues[18] published an extensive review of 111 patients who underwent placement of 706 implants in conjunction with a variety of flap reconstructions, including bone flaps, but HBO therapy was not available. They noted an increased failure rate in those patients who had received radiation, but their overall integration rate was 92.9%. In addition to numerous findings and recommendations, they recommended waiting 12 months before implant placement and allowing double the normal time for osseointegration. Teoh and colleagues[19] specifically addressed implants placed in the microvascular fibula flap and found that patients who had received radiation therapy before implant placement had a lower implant survival rate compared with those who did not (92% vs 99%). They also noted a higher failure rate in those patients with a previous history of HBO therapy and attributed it to their small sample size. Smolka and colleagues[20] also demonstrated the high success rate (92%) for implants placed in the fibula. In their study, 85% of the patients had a history of radiation therapy, and they did not find any correlation with failure. Some investigators have also suggested an improved rate of integration in postirradiated flap reconstructions versus implants placed in nonvascularized bone grafts. An animal study, which has not been replicated in clinical trials, demonstrated that radiated vascularized bone flaps healed better than radiated nonvascularized bone flaps.[21] Other investigators have suggested that osseointegration may be more successful with certain vascularized bone flaps. With regard to the fibula flap, this may be secondary to the quantity of cortical bone available in this flap.[18,19] Although none of these case series can conclusively answer the question of the need for HBO therapy before implant placement in free tissue flaps, taken together, they confirm the feasibility of dental implant placement without HBO therapy, which has been reported by many surgeons.

Regardless of opposing viewpoints on HBO therapy, surgeons agree that the irradiated site presents obstacles to integration and long-term maintenance of dental implants, but irradiation should not preclude the placement of implants. Factors to consider include the dose of radiation received at the site of planned placement. For example, the anterior mandible often is spared in the treatment of many head and neck cancers and does not receive more than 50 Gy. In addition, newer technology, such as intensity modulated radiation therapy, may spare larger areas from receiving full doses of radiation. Location of implantation should also be considered. Poor bone quality in the posterior maxilla may contribute to poor integration rates seen after radiation, and the effect may be additive. Treatment plans that focus on placement of fixtures in the anterior maxilla take advantage of better bone quality and the fact that this site often receives less radiation. Mention should also be made of alternative medical therapies used to improve healing after radiation therapy, including the use of vitamin E and pentoxifylline, which have been demonstrated to improve soft tissue healing after radiation therapy and may likewise improve bone healing.[22,23] Finally, some investigators have suggested that immediate placement of dental implants at the time of reconstruction allows integration before radiation therapy and eliminates the question of HBO therapy altogether.

Immediate Versus Delayed Implant Placement

Implant placement can be performed simultaneously with the primary reconstruction or delayed as a secondary procedure after healing of the flap and completion of any indicated adjuvant therapy, such as radiation treatment. Investigators have reported successful outcomes with dental implants placed at the time of tumor ablation and reconstruction, as well as with delayed placement of fixtures.[24,25] Proponents of each technique offer advantages and disadvantages. Immediate placement of dental implants at the time of free flap reconstruction offers several advantages. Patients are restored faster and are not subjected to an additional procedure for placement of the implants. Some investigators have also suggested a higher probability for successful integration, if the implants are placed at the time of the initial reconstruction and radiation is delayed for 6 weeks after reconstruction.[24] They propose that if the patient is to be irradiated, implant integration is more likely to be successful if the implants are placed before the bone flap (neomandible) is exposed to radiation.[24] Despite this hypothesis, Fenlon and collegues[26] compared immediate versus delayed (3 months) placement and found a significant loss of one-third of implants placed in before irradiation. They did not comment on the time span between placement and commencement of irradiation. Significantly, they also reported that one-fifth of immediate-placement implants were unusable and another one-third were suboptimal for prosthetic rehabilitation. Early reports recommended placing the implants before positioning the flap in its final position, that is, on the side table or before disconnecting the pedicle. Although this recommendation may make placement easier and in the later case decrease ischemic time, implants often end up in unusable positions, either placed far too buccal or lingual. Other investigators have suggested improved positioning when the implants are placed after the flap is in its final position. This placement may allow more accurate orientation of the implants. Immediate placement also adds to the time the patient is under anesthesia, which can add to the risk of lengthy surgery. Hirsch and colleagues[27] have described a technique using stereolithography and virtual surgery to prefabricate surgical guides that can then be used intraoperatively for contouring bone flaps and placing dental implants. This technique allows exceptional accuracy in translating the preoperative plan to the operating room and holds promise in decreasing surgical time while allowing accurate configuration of the neomandible and positioning of dental implants (**Fig. 3**).

Delayed placement overcomes some of these shortcomings but does lengthen treatment time. An important advantage of delayed placement of implants is the opportunity that it provides the prosthodontist to assess the exact needs for reconstruction and make recommendations for placement.[20] Finally, if the reconstruction is for oncologic reasons, some consideration must be given to prognosis of the patient. It is important to match reconstructive efforts to prognosis, and this is especially true regarding dental implants. Many patients requiring composite resections for malignant tumors have poor survival rates, and immediate reconstruction with dental implants may not be indicated. Garrett and colleagues[28] reported a significant loss in number of patients undergoing dental implant rehabilitation after oncologic resections of the mandible and questioned the practice of immediate placement at the time of primary reconstruction. In addition, immediate placement adds to the complexity and risks of the reconstruction, including the potential for infection, and delay of adjuvant therapies, such as irradiation.

At present, it is the authors' opinion that the advantages and predictability of delayed placement outweigh those of immediate placement in most cases. If delayed placement is planned, there remains the question of how much delay. A definitive answer is not available, but several investigators have made suggestions based on their experience. Jacobson and colleagues[29] recommended waiting for at least 1 year, based on several factors, including likelihood of disease control and improved healing, as the patients improve their nutrition and overall well-being. In the aforementioned study by Garrett and colleagues,[28] patient enrollment took significantly longer than anticipated in response to patient's desires to delay implant placement, having already gone through extensive ablative and reconstructive surgeries.

Waiting for a minimum of 12 months in most cases is recommended, but exceptions are made based on the unique circumstances of each case. Consideration should also be given to obtaining any indicated surveillance imaging, such as positron emission tomography, before any flap revision (see later discussion) of implant placement because surgical maneuvers can cloud the interpretation of these studies.

SOFT TISSUE

Ideally, a dental implant should emerge through a band of immobile, keratinized mucosa. This process allows for healthy peri-implant tissues that are resistant to bacterial invasion and peri-implantitis. The ideal thickness of tissue around an implant should be less than 3 mm, because thickness greater than 4 mm creates a noncleansable deep pocket. Although controversy exists whether or not keratinized tissue is needed around implants in patients having undergone reconstruction with free tissue transfer, one can see the direct benefit of having the keratinized tissue as part of what is expected in these patients; these tissues are more resistant to abrasion, which is good for oral hygiene. But tissues imported from distant sites

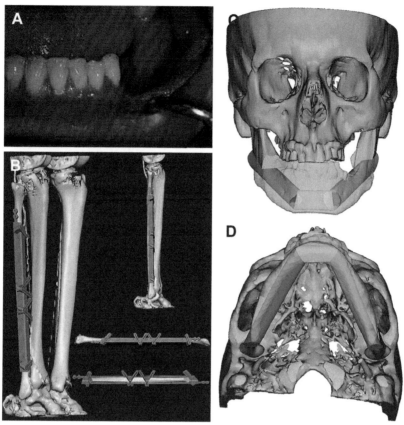

Fig. 3. (*A*) Fibula osteocutaneous flap placed too far laterally. (*B*) Preoperative planning using virtual surgery and stereolithography for fabrication of an osteotomy guide for accurate fibula shaping. (*C*, *D*) Virtual surgical planning to ensure proper shape and placement of fibula in neomandible in relation to maxilla.

do not satisfy these requirements. At the time of reconstruction, the main goal is obtaining a good seal and preventing the development of oral-cutaneous fistulae. Soft tissue components of free tissue flaps are usually thick and mobile, whereas their cutaneous component lacks the characteristics of keratinized mucosa (**Fig. 4**). In addition, they are often insensate to varying degrees allowing trauma to go undetected. Implants emerging through these thick soft tissue paddles are almost invariably affected by peri-implantitis. They are difficult to keep clean, and this often results in chronically inflamed and exuberant tissue. If the tissue has been irradiated, it is usually atrophic and even less resistant to trauma from prostheses and peri-implantitis. In addition to these shortcomings related to implants, the thick soft tissue lacks support for the prosthesis. Removable prosthesis requires a stable base, and the thick, mobile tissue associated with most free flaps does not provide it. Various techniques are recommended to overcome this "pillow" effect. Techniques described later can be used to thin the flap. Alternatively,

Panagos and Hirsch[30] have described a technique using zygomatic (long) implants placed through the radial forearm flap to offer support and retention to a maxillary denture. This technique can

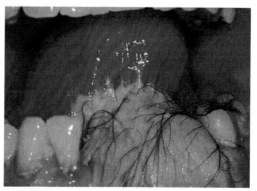

Fig. 4. Radial forearm fasciocutaneous flap provides mobility to tongue after reconstruction for a defect in the anterior floor of mouth, but its position over the alveolus precludes prosthetic rehabilitation without modification.

help in overcoming the pliability of the flap, which results in displacement of the prosthesis. Most flaps, however, require modification of the soft tissue.

The most common problems with soft tissue are thickness and lack of a vestibule, which can be addressed in several ways. The soft tissue can be thinned aggressively using an open or closed technique. A flap can be developed in a subdermal plane, and it can be aggressively defatted and repositioned. Alternatively, aggressive liposuction can be performed on the flap. The cannula can also be turned toward the dermis (opposite to traditional liposuction) and can serve to depilate the flap if hair growth is a problem (**Fig. 5**). Over the alveolus, the skin flap can be removed in a supraperiosteal plane. A split-thickness skin graft can be placed or the wound can be left to heal by secondary intention. A prefabricated splint is fixed in place for 1 to 2 weeks to aid in healing (**Fig. 6**). Ideally, a vestibule depth of 1.0 to 1.5 cm is ideal.[31] If the skin paddle is to be preserved and depends on a septocutanoeus perforator, this should be taken into account. Neovascularization occurs to a variable degree in free tissue transfer, and the skin paddle often remains dependent on its perforator. A handheld doppler probe can be used to identify its location before manipulation, although this is not considered to be an issue. If additional hard tissue grafting is indicated, it should be done first, and soft tissue refinement should be delayed until the secondary bone grafting has healed (see later discussion on bone techniques). If bone union is present, remaining hardware is removed to avoid problems with implant site preparation later. There is some evidence that the soft tissue component of free flaps undergoes some adaptation after placement of prosthesis (**Fig. 7**). This process has been described by Kovács[32] as "adaptive rebuilding," who found that peri-implantitis and pocket depths reduced over time.

BONE TECHNIQUES

Continuity defects of the mandible resulting from oncologic resections are most commonly reconstructed immediately with vascularized bone-containing flaps, which include a soft tissue component (osseocutaneous or myo-osseous).[2,20,24] Large avulsive traumatic injuries involving the mandible and large (>5 cm) benign defects of the anterior mandible are most reliably reconstructed with vascularized bone.[1] In 1989, Hidalgo[33] introduced the fibula free flap for mandibular reconstruction, and it quickly became the reconstruction workhorse of continuity defects. Alternative bone-containing

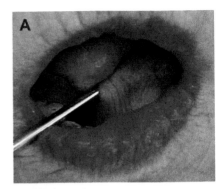
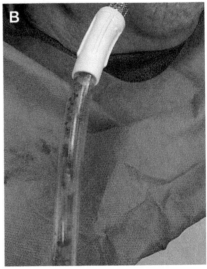

Fig. 5. (A) Liposuction performed on bulky radial forearm flap after healing. Cannula opening is turned in the traditional manner away from dermis and also toward dermis. (B) Aggressive liposuction can yield a surprising amount of fat in many flaps and may be all that is necessary.

vascularized flaps include the iliac crest deep circumflex iliac artery (DCIA), scapula, and radial forearm. Each flap has its own merits and disadvantages. Despite the ability of these flaps to reestablish continuity of the mandible, dental rehabilitation is challenging and typically requires the placement of endosseous implants either in the native mandible or neomandible or both for a satisfactory prosthesis. Each bone-containing flap offers variable bone quality and quantity and specific considerations for implant placement. With regard to implant placement and vascularized bone flaps, the mandible has been more widely studied than the maxilla and is discussed first.

The most common criticism of free tissue bone flaps is the amount of bone stock available and its shape (**Fig. 8**). Depending on the amount of bone removed, all current bone flaps usually require some osteotomies to recapitulate the

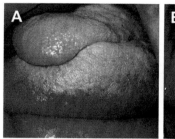
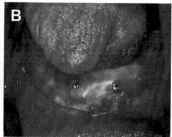

Fig. 6. (*A, B*) Bulky flap used in reconstructing anterior floor of mouth and interfering with fabrication of prosthesis. Flap is thinned aggressively using an open approach, and a prefabricated splint is placed and secured with screws or circummandibular wires.

shape of the mandible (**Fig. 9**). Positioning of the bone requires balancing prosthodontic needs with esthetic requirements for flap contouring and placement. For example, if the reconstruction involves the anterior mandible in the edentulous patient, the neomandible should be positioned slightly lingual in the anterior to avoid the pseudo-class III relationship to the maxilla.[20]

At present, the most commonly used bone-containing flaps to reconstruct the mandible are the fibula (vascularized fibula osteocutaneous free flap) and the radius (radial forearm osteocutaneous free flap). Less commonly used flaps are the iliac crest (DCIA) flap and the scapula free flap. A general rule is that 5.0 to 5.75 × 10 mm of bone is necessary to accept dental implants. Frodel and colleagues[34] and Moscoso and colleagues[35] have demonstrated that the bone stock available from most fibulas is adequate for dental implant placement, while the radius was the least implantable of all bone-containing flaps. Although some investigators have demonstrated that implants can be placed into the radius, it is rarely practical without additional grafting.[36] The iliac crest free (DCIA) flap provides the most bone stock for dental implant reconstruction. The morbidity associated with its harvest, is a disadvantage and has

limited its use. The scapula is highly variable in the quantity and quality of bone that it provides. It is usually used only when large, independent skin paddles are needed, that is, for through-and-through defects that involve the mandible.

Based on its reliable anatomy, ease of harvest, and bone stock, the fibula has become the most popular free bone flap for reconstruction of mandibular continuity defects in most centers. In addition, it has been the most widely studied bone flap with regard to dental implant placement. Implant survival rates for those placed in the fibula approach those placed in native mandible. Teoh and colleagues[19] reported cumulative survival rates for implants placed in the fibula to be 97%, 97%, and 79.9% at 1, 5, and 10 years, respectively. This rate included implants in patients who

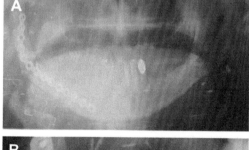

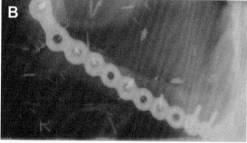

Fig. 8. (*A*) Panorex radiograph demonstrating bone height of fibula flap compared with native dentate mandible. (*B*) Panorex radiograph demonstrating bone height of radial forearm osteocutaneous flap compared with dentate mandible.

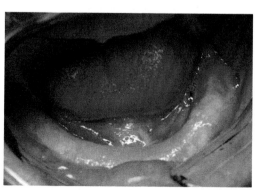

Fig. 7. Adaptive remodeling of fibula skin paddle resulting from denture wear only.

A

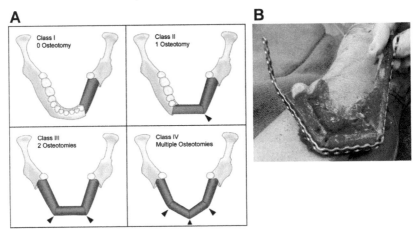

B

Fig. 9. (*A*) Simple osteotomy designs allow recapitulation of satisfactory mandibular contours in most cases. (*From* Smolka K, Kraehenbuehl M, Eggensperger N, et al. Fibula free flap reconstruction of the mandible in cancer patients: evaluation of a combined surgical and prosthodontic treatment concept. Oral Oncol 2008;44(6):573; with permission.) (*B*) Typically the anterior male mandible can be addressed with 2 osteotomies in the fibula.

succumbed to disease and those lost to follow-up and was in concordance with success rates of 92% at 9 years, published by Smolka and colleagues.[20] The length of the fibula allows reconstruction of total mandibulectomies, and it has a thick cortex, which allows bicortical engagement of the implants.

Although the fibula's height of 13 to 15 mm approximates the height of an edentulous mandible, the dentate mandible can present problems. If the flap is located flush with the inferior border of the mandible, the restoring team should expect to use tissue extension abutments to bring implants to higher levels and possibly the fabrication of a suprastructure, with the added disadvantages of additional cost and complexity (**Fig. 10**). Also, it can result in a long moment arm and increased lateral forces on the implants. Numerous modifications of the technique to overcome some of the limitations of the bone stock with the fibula have been developed. The "double-barrell" fibula flap was described by

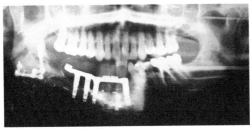

Fig. 10. Suprastructure placed after implant placement in a fibula flap to overcome height discrepancy.

Horiuchi and colleagues.[37] In this case, an intervening segment of fibula is removed, allowing the fibula to be folded on itself to provide more height. Folding the flap does put the pedicle at some risk for kinking or compression, and the benefit is questionable. Distraction osteogenesis has also been used to improve the height of the fibula, but recent reports have demonstrated that the technique is not without complications (**Fig. 11**).[38] Despite the availability of these techniques, the most efficacious technique is likely simply placing the fibula near the superior border of the residual native mandible (**Fig. 12**). If the graft was located flush with the superior border of the mandible, the restoring team should be able to fabricate more favorable restorations and potentially incurring in less cost. Although this process can lead to some contour discrepancy along the jaw line, it is usually less noticeable than expected, and remodeling results in a satisfactory result more often than not (**Fig. 13**).[20] In addition, if unacceptable to the patient, it is often easier to augment the inferior border because there is less risk for graft exposure to the oral cavity and less soft tissues contraction leading to resorbtion.

Augmentation of the bone stock can be performed as a primary or secondary procedure. Often, a portion of the bone flap is discarded while contouring, which can be morselized in a bone mill and placed at the junction of the flap and the native mandible at the osteotomy sites. Caution should be exercised if radiation therapy is planned because this nonvascularized free bone component of the reconstruction may not have time to heal and may lead to a nidus for wound breakdown

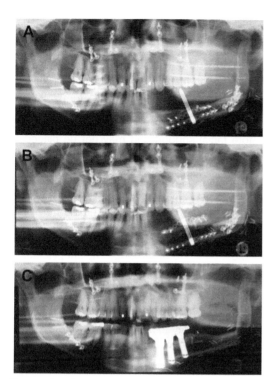

Fig. 11. (*A–C*) Distraction osteogenesis of fibula flap to increase height for placement of dental implants near the superior border. (*Courtesy of* Eric J. Dierks, DMD, MD, FACS, Portland, OR.)

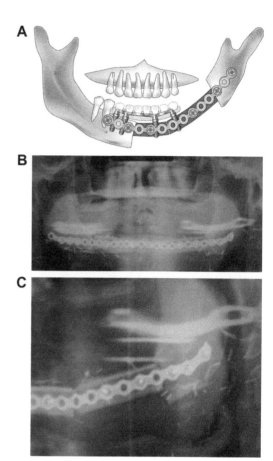

Fig. 12. (*A–C*) Schematic demonstrating placement of the fibula construct near the superior border to decrease long moment arms and need for extensive suprastructures. (*From* Smolka K, Kraehenbuehl M, Eggensperger N, et al. Fibula free flap reconstruction of the mandible in cancer patients: evaluation of a combined surgical and prosthodontic treatment concept. Oral Oncol 2008;44(6):574; with permission.)

and infection, which can delay initiation of radiation therapy. Allograft can also be placed along the cut surface of the radial forearm osteocutaneous flap to augment it. Bone morphogenic protein is gaining popularity as a graft material for maxillofacial applications, but it should not be placed at the time of primary reconstruction in oncologic resections secondary to concerns regarding potential stimulation of residual tumor cells. It can be considered in secondary grafting or in cases of benign disease.

Patients undergoing prosthetic rehabilitation with dental implants should be aware that there will be multiple surgical procedures, including the primary reconstruction with free tissue transfer, revision and debulking of soft tissues, implant placement, and restorative phase. It requires a significant commitment from the patient with regard to time and energy. Postoperative prosthetic workup before implant placement is must. A decision must be established regarding the type of prosthesis used, such as fixed, removable, or hybrid. The prosthetic phase starts at the initial consultation and subsequent surgical interventions and continues with the fabrication of wax trial denture for evaluation of proper soft and hard tissue support, function, and esthetics. When acceptable

results have been achieved, this trial denture is duplicated as a surgical template for implant placement. Cone beam computed tomography, implant planning software, and steriolithographic models allow precise planning and decrease the risk of improper placement. Implants should be placed 1.5 to 2 mm away from existing teeth, and if no teeth are present the implants should have 3-mm interval between one another. Often it is best to avoid sites of previous osteotomies in the bone flap or native bone because fibrous tissue may be present along with incomplete ossification. The number of implants depends on the type of continuity defect and whether the patient is totally or partially edentulous.

To satisfy the prosthetic requirements of support, stability, and retention, at least 2 direct

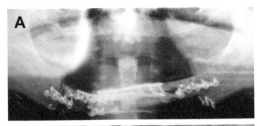

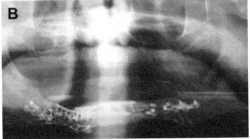

Fig. 13. (*A, B*) Remodeling of fibula flap placed in dentate mandible at the time of resection and after remodeling.

attachments or 4 fixtures for the bar overdenture are indicated. The minimum amount of interocclusal height for such an option should be no less than 12 mm or 15 mm from the bone level to the occlusal plane of the arch to be restored.[39] The implant-fixed retained prosthesis requires a minimum of 5 implants between the mental foramina, with a distal cantilever off of each side that replaces the posterior teeth. This process is the classic BrÅnemark approach and requires good anteroposterior location of the flap in relationship to the maxillary arch so as not to create long horizontal cantilevers due to misalignment of the graft with the opposing arch. In addition, the implants should not be placed in a straight line. They should have an adequate anteroposterior distance within a taper or a square arch configuration.

Implants placed after free tissue transfer for reconstruction of maxillary defects have not been as well studied as the mandible. Obturators are still commonly used to rehabilitate patients with maxillectomy defects. In addition, maxillary defects related to oncologic resections are less common than those involving the mandible. For these reasons, the maxilla has not received the same amount of attention. At present, an increasing number of maxillary defects are being primarily reconstructed with both soft tissue and bone-containing flaps. Prosthodontic requirements for the maxilla differ in many aspects from the mandible, but some of the same limitations regarding free flaps apply. There are maneuvers to overcome these shortcomings.

Unlike the mandible in which the fibula has taken on a preeminent reconstructive role in most cases, a wider variety of flaps are promoted by different surgeons for reconstructing maxillary defects. Often there is a need for greater latitude with the soft tissue component of the flap to enable separation of nasal, sinal, oral, and sometimes cranial cavities. Bone is often used to restore facial support and may not be placed in a position that is suitable for implants. Because the maxilla offers a more stable base for prosthodontics than the mandible, it offers more latitude with options for dental implant placement. Implants placed in the residual maxilla may offer enough support for the entire prosthesis. Similar to the mandible, the iliac crest free flap offers the most bone stock for dental implant placement in the maxilla. When using the iliac crest free flap in the maxilla, donor site morbidity and the need for vein grafts limit its use. The fibula offers good bone stock, but the skin paddle is bulky and limited in its ability to be adjusted. The radial forearm osseocutaneous flap offers excellent soft tissue options, but the bone stock is poor. It is possible, however, to use the radius in many cases as a strut to support a denture, especially if combined with dental implants placed in the residual maxilla.[40]

Placement of additional corticocancellous grafts along with the initial flap is often precluded by communication with the sinus. Secondary bone-grafting techniques are often more reliable. The iliac crest or tibia serve as potential donor sites for cancellous grafts to augment the bone.

FUTURE DIRECTIONS

The future holds promise for additional advancements and refinements in combining free tissue transfer and dental implants. A technique that has been published uses free transfer of a portion of the femur to reconstruct isolated alveolar defects using an intraoral anastomosis and avoids a cervical incision.[41] Progress is being made in developing a reliable replacement for oral mucosa that perhaps could be substituted for the skin component of current free flaps to provide a more favorable environment for peri-implant.[42] Prefabricated flaps built on implanted frameworks based on the perforator-flap concept may overcome some of the issues with bone quantity and shape. Perhaps, implants will be placed within these frameworks, allowing transplant of a hard and soft tissue flap containing integrated implants.

Although the ultimate goal of a functional and esthetic dental rehabilitation after oncologic resection and reconstruction seems intuitive, quality-of-life studies have not demonstrated a distinct advantage in patients undergoing implant placement. This advantage could be secondary to the enormous amount of time and effort involved in these complex treatments. Although cost is a significant barrier to dental implant placement in many cases, studies involving patients in which cost is not an issue (implants and prostheses are provided free to the patient) still demonstrated a remarkable number of patients choosing not to undergo dental rehabilitation. Teoh and colleagues[19] reported that only 29 of 260 patients (11.2%) who underwent microvascular reconstruction of the mandible received dental implants. Similar results were reported by Garrett and colleagues,[28] who reported a significant delay in prosthetic rehabilitation and significant attrition in their study. A variety of reasons were cited, including poor prognosis, systemic disease, and time commitment. The oncologic patient is often psychologically and physically spent after undergoing multimodality therapy and is not interested in pursuing further surgery. Also, many abuse tobacco and have multiple medical comorbidities that decrease successful rehabilitation with osseointegrated implant prosthetics. Despite the promise of full dental rehabilitation offered by present technology, more work is needed to establish selection criteria and determine who benefits most from dental implants, who should receive them, and when is the most appropriate time for placement.

SUMMARY

Aside from the significant potential for disfigurement, disabilities resulting from composite defects of the oral cavity include impaired speech, swallowing, and mastication and compromised control of saliva. Although microvascular techniques have given the surgeon several choices for replacing bone and soft tissue, there remain significant challenges to rehabilitating the patient to a functioning occlusion that allows unencumbered mastication and articulation and provides adequate esthetics. Endosseous implants often provide the best opportunity to achieve a successful prosthetic rehabilitation. Current reconstructive techniques, however, rarely provide an ideal site for implant placement, and site preparation techniques are required to modify the flap and provide an integrated implant in proper position that can be maintained long term.

REFERENCES

1. Foster RD, Anthony JP, Sharma A. Vascularized bone flaps versus nonvascularized bone grafts for mandibular reconstruction: an outcome analysis of primary bony union and endosseous implant success. Head Neck 1999;21(1):66–71.
2. Rosenthal EL, Dixon SF. Free flap complications: when is enough, enough? Curr Opin Otolaryngol Head Neck Surg 2003;11(4):236–9.
3. Desjardins RP. Occlusal considerations for the partial mandibulectomy patient. J Prosthet Dent 1979;41(3):308–15.
4. Teng MS, Futran ND. Osteoradionecrosis of the mandible. Curr Opin Otolaryngol Head Neck Surg 2005;13(4):217–21.
5. Bennett MH, Feldmeier J, Hampson N, et al. Hyperbaric oxygen for late radiation injury. [review]. Cochrane Database Syst Rev 2007;(2):1–26.
6. Marx RE. A new concept in the treatment of osteoradionecrosis. J Oral Maxillofac Surg 1983; 41(6):351–7.
7. Marx RE. Osteoradionecrosis: a new concept of its pathophysiology. J Oral Maxillofac Surg 1983; 41(5):283–8.
8. Marx RE, Johnson RP, Kline SN. Prevention of osteoradionecrosis: a randomized prospective clinical trial of hyperbaric oxygen versus penicillin. J Am Dent Assoc 1985;111(1):49–54.
9. Annane D, Depondt J, Aubert P, et al. Hyperbaric oxygen therapy for radionecrosis of the jaw: a randomized, placebo-controlled, double blind trial from the ORN96 group. J Clin Oncol 2004;22(24): 4893–900.
10. Gal TJ, Yueh B, Futran ND. Influence of prior hyperbaric oxygen therapy in complications following microvascular reconstruction for advanced osteoradionecrosis. Arch Otolaryngol Head Neck Surg 2003;129(1):72–6.
11. Granstrom G. Radiotherapy, osseointegration and hyperbaric oxygen therapy. Periodontol 2000 2003; 33:145–62.
12. Eckert SE, Desjardins RP, Keller EE, et al. Endosseous implants in an irradiated tissue bed. J Prosthet Dent 1996;76(1):45–9.
13. Wagner W, Esser E, Ostkamp K. Osseointegration of dental implants in patients with and without radiotherapy. Acta Oncol 1998;37(7–8):693–6.
14. Schoen PJ, Raghoeber GM, Bouma J, et al. Rehabilitation of oral function in head and neck cancer patients after radiotherapy with implant retained dentures: effects of hyperbaric oxygen therapy. Oral Oncol 2007;43(4):379–88.
15. Granstrom G. Placement of dental implants in irradiated bone: the case for using hyperbaric oxygen. J Oral Maxillofac Surg 2006;64(5):812–8.
16. Donoff RB. Treatment of the irradiated patient with dental implants: the case against hyperbaric oxygen treatment. J Oral Maxillofac Surg 2006;64(5):819–22.
17. Esposito M, Grusovin MG, Patel S, et al. Interventions for replacing missing teeth: hyperbaric oxygen

therapy for irradiated patients who require dental implants. Cochrane Database Syst Rev 2008;4:1–14.

18. Cuesta-Gil M, Caicoya SO, Riba-Garcia F, et al. Oral rehabilitation with osseointegrated implants in oncologic patients. J Oral Maxillofac Surg 2009;67(11): 2485–96.

19. Teoh KH, Huryn JM, Patel S, et al. Implant prosthodontic rehabilitation of fibula free-flap reconstructed mandibles: a Memorial Sloan-Kettering Cancer Center review of prognostic factors and implant outcomes. Int J Oral Maxillofac Implants 2005; 20(5):738–46.

20. Smolka K, Kraehenbuehl M, Eggensperger N, et al. Fibula free flap reconstruction of the mandible in cancer patients: evaluation of a combined surgical and prosthodontic treatment concept. Oral Oncol 2008;44(6):571–81.

21. Evans HB, Brown S, Hurst LN. The effects of early postoperative radiation on vascularized bone grafts. Ann Plast Surg 1991;26(6):505–10.

22. Futran ND, Trotti A, Gwede C. Pentoxifylline in the treatment of radiation-related soft tissue injury: preliminary observations. Laryngoscope 1997; 107(3):391–5.

23. Delanian S, Porcher R, Balla-Mekias S, et al. Randomized, placebo-controlled trial of combined pentoxifylline and tocopherol for regression of superficial radiation-induced fibrosis. Br J Radiol 2003;21(13):2545–50.

24. Urken ML, Buchbinder D, Costantino PD, et al. Oromandibular reconstruction using microvascular composite flaps. Arch Otolaryngol Head Neck Surg 1998;124(1):46–55.

25. Kildal M, Wei F, Chang Y, et al. Mandibular reconstruction with fibula osteoseptocutaneous free flap and osseointegrated dental implants. Clin Plast Surg 2001;28(2):403–10.

26. Fenlon MR, Lyons A, Farrell S, et al. Factors affecting survival and usefulness of implants placed in vascularized free composite grafts used in head and neck cancer reconstruction. Clin Implant Dent Relat Res 2009. [Epub ahead of print].

27. Hirsch DL, Garfein ES, Christensen AM, et al. Use of computer aided design and computer aided manufacturing to produce orthognathically ideal surgical outcomes: a paradigm shift in head and neck reconstruction. J Oral Maxillofac Surg 2009; 67(10):2115–22.

28. Garrett N, Roumanas ED, Blackwell KE, et al. Efficacy of conventional and implant-supported mandibular resection prostheses: study overview and treatment options. J Prosthet Dent 2006;96(1):13–24.

29. Jacobson M, Tjellstrom A, Albrektsson T, et al. Integration of titanium implants in irradiated bone. Histologic and clinical study. Ann Otol Rhinol Laryngol 1988;97(4 Pt 1):337–40.

30. Panagos P, Hirsch DL. Resection of a large, central hemangioma with reconstruction using a radial forearm flap combined with zygomatic and pterygoid implants. J Oral Maxillofac Surg 2009;67(3):630–6.

31. Martin JW, Lemon J, Schusterman M. Oral and dental rehabilitation after mandible reconstruction. Operat Tech Plast Resconstr Surg 1996;3(4):264–71.

32. Kovács AF. The fate of osseointegrated implants in patients following oral cancer surgery and mandibular reconstruction. Head Neck 2000;22(2):111–9.

33. Hidalgo DA. Fibula free flap: a new method of mandible reconstruction. Plast Reconstr Surg 1989;84(1):71–9.

34. Frodel JL, Funk GF, Capper DT, et al. Osseointegrated implants: a comparative study of bone thickness in four vascularized bone flaps. Plast Reconstr Surg 1993;92(3):449–55.

35. Moscoso JF, Keller J, Genden E, et al. Vascularized bone flaps in oromandibular reconstruction. A comparative anatomic study of bone stock from various donor sites to assess suitability for enosseous dental implants. Arch Otolaryngol Head Neck Surg 1994;120(1):36–43.

36. Martin IC, Cawood JI, Vaughan ED, et al. Endosseous implants in the irradiated composite radial forearm free flap. Int J Oral Maxillofac Surg 1992; 21(5):266–70.

37. Horiuchi K, Hattori A, Inada I, et al. Mandibular reconstruction using the double barrel fibular graft. Microsurgery 1995;16(7):450–4.

38. Lizio G, Corinaldesi G, Pieri F, et al. problems with dental implants that were placed on vertically distracted fibular free flaps after resection: a report of six cases. Br J Oral Maxillofac Surg 2009;47(6): 455–60.

39. Misch CE. Dental implant prosthetics. Mandibular full-arch implant fixed prosthetic option. Philadelphia (PA): Mosby; 2005. p. 252–60. Chapter 16.

40. Villaret DB, Futran NA. The indications and outcomes in the use of osteocutaneous radial forearm free flap 2003;25(6):475–81.

41. Gaggl AJ, Bürger HK, Chiari FM. Free microvascular transfer of segmental corticocancellous femur for reconstruction of the alveolar ridge. Br J Oral Maxillofac Surg 2008;46(3):211–7.

42. Moharamzadeh K, Brook IM, Van Noort R, et al. Tissue engineered oral mucosa: a review of the scientific literature. J Dent Res 2007;86(2):115–24.

Retrieval and Analysis of Explanted and In Situ Implants Including Bone Grafts

Jack E. Lemons, PhD

KEYWORDS

- Retrieval and analysis • Dental implants
- Histology histomorphometry

INTRODUCTION
Brief History

The retrieval and analysis of surgical implant devices as an integral component of academic research was expanded in the United States after an initial cosponsored consensus conference in the 1970s.[1] Guidelines developed at that meeting progressed to more standardized procedures, thereby permitting data exchanges at multiple levels within the profession.[2,3] Subsequent consensus conferences expanded the details of information to be collected and clearly demonstrated the values of multidisciplinary studies for improving existing and developing new devices and procedures to enhance clinical outcomes associated with surgical implant devices.[4–6]

In Vitro Plus Laboratory and Human Specimens

Most implant device–oriented research, development, and applications initiate from an idea and in vitro laboratory studies to determine the physical, mechanical, chemical, electrical, and biologic (biocompatibility) properties of a device. In each situation, these studies are specific for the proposed clinical application. This is done to determine the initial safety of the intended clinical applications. Subsequent directed studies to evaluate efficacy extend to laboratory in vivo simulations for host biocompatibility interactions that includes function and preliminary human clinical

trials that are based on detailed protocols developed from the prior studies. One benefit of human retrieval and analysis (revision surgery or post mortem) investigations is the opportunity to compare, retrospectively, the pre- and postconditions of the device and host environment, including information from the actual human applications. This has been a theme within most device and retrieval programs and these types of programs now exist throughout the world.

Local Experience Since the 1970s

The program (University of Alabama at Birmingham [UAB]) discussed in this article was initiated in the early 1970s. The central theme was to investigate tissue and device interfaces and the conditions of transfers specific to synthetic origin elements from the device (biomaterials) and associated forces from the host associated with device function (biomechanics). This program was jointly based on UAB's schools of dentistry, medicine, and engineering and from the outset was interdisciplinary. It was realized that factors from patients, the technology of surgery and restoration, and the device should be separated using the expertise from those trained in the biologic, clinical, and physical sciences. This team concept was carried forward to regular meetings of all involved. The central foci of these meetings have been what has caused the need for this revision surgery (removal of the device) and what might have

Departments of Prosthodontics, Surgery and Biomedical Engineering, Schools of Dentistry, Medicine and Engineering, University of Alabama at Birmingham, 1530 Third Avenue South, SDB Box 61, Birmingham, AL 35294-0007, USA
E-mail address: jack.lemons@ortho.uab.edu

Oral Maxillofacial Surg Clin N Am 22 (2010) 419–423
doi:10.1016/j.coms.2010.06.002

been done to minimize this type of clinical outcome.

It was recognized that observations on the devices per se could be reported with confidence; however, overall cause-effect relationships often required testing of hypotheses. We called this approach forensic discovery. Over time and experience, thousands of specimens have been collected, leading to graduate student MS and PhD theses and dissertations, resident-based studies, and investigations focused on interests of faculty members. Often, studies have been based on single observations or, confirming or not, observations of others. In all situations, a concern has been the statistical significance from a clinical perspective, especially related to the numerator (number studied) versus the denominator (number used clinically). Specific to device properties, multiple examples exist where studies based on retrieval and analysis have confirmed that an initial observation would result in expanded interactions and, in some cases, these represented a larger number (thousands of devices). Thereby the overall outcome was a circumstance of statistical and clinical significance.

Current and Future Opportunities

As discussed previously, recognition of value associated with appropriate studies of explanted and in situ postmortem surgical implant devices has resulted in expansion of national and international programs. Another aspect is the opportunity to combine with existing and evolving clinical registries concerned with device outcomes, which should further enhance correlations of device-specific studies with expanded and detailed clinical records. We anticipate the evolution of regional, national, and international networks for information exchange based on secure Internet and Web systems. Key to this approach will be exchanges earlier in the cycles of device clinical applications while protecting the rights of all stakeholders.

MATERIALS AND METHODS
Summary of Experience for Identifying, Removing, Transferring, Receiving, Recording, Analyzing, and Reporting for Different Sources and Types of Specimens

Retrieved implant specimens for detailed analyses have originated from several sources. Studies of the preclinical specimens from university-based laboratory in vitro and in vivo investigations have provided the instrumentation, techniques, and experience for subsequent analyses. Human specimens from revision surgeries include devices that are removed and replaced by another device and are called clinical failures. In contrast, those from postmortem donors that are in situ at the time of donation are called clinical successes. To analyze and compare results, records and details are obtained from protocols based on national and international standards.[2,3]

In clinic-to-laboratory transfers, specimens are normally placed in containers with 10% buffered formalin, following procedures similar to tissue processing for pathology studies. At UAB, device specimens are transferred through the Department of Pathology, and retrieval and analysis programs treat the device as one part of evaluations (physical aspects of the device) needed to enhance patient care. All aspects of study fall under institutional review board (IRB)–and Health Insurance Portability and Accountability Act (HIPPA)–approved protocols. Off-site specimens must also include patient and clinician approvals for studies plus nationally approved packaging and transferring procedures. The UAB program has developed a minimum data set (a form) for information to be collected and transferred with each "general" type of specimen. On receipt, all specimens are initially treated as contaminated by infectious agents and all handling is conducted to assure safety and no or minimal damage to avoid altering as-received device and tissue conditions. This step often requires information exchange with the clinical investigator. To assure confidentiality, all explanted specimens are identified with a code IXXX with sequential numbering. After careful and appropriate observation and removal of loose debris, the specimens move to a triage step where they are separated into tiers I, II or III. Most specimens that are tier I represent conditions where all observations are "as anticipated" and specimens are moved to secure storage; tiers II and III are when something "unanticipated" is noted and these specimens are transferred to a group meeting for more detailed considerations.

The group meeting includes all interested parties where students include undergraduate and graduate levels, clinical residents, staff, and faculty. All meet together to observe and comment. The clinical participants present the patient and treatment information (including available radiology and pathology studies) whereas the nonclinical participants present the physical (engineering) aspects of the device and associated instrumentation. These discussions often result in hypotheses about what might have caused the unanticipated features and what studies might provide answers. Protocols, studies, and peer-reviewed publications develop from this initial step. Tier II represents unanticipated alterations of the device, tissues, or related information where specimens are judged not to have influenced the clinical outcome. Tier III represents the more in-depth studies where the device or associated technology could have influenced the need for revision surgery. One special aspect of device and tissue studies related to biomaterial and biomechanical properties is the extensive instrumentation, test machine, and analytical analysis systems required to develop quantitative data. Additionally, because studies often focus on the implant-to-tissue interface, a fully equipped histology/histomorphometry laboratory, including nondecalcified and implant sectioning (Exakt) equipment, has developed to evaluate these types of specimens.

Postmortem en bloc device and host tissue specimens from individuals donating for research have provided opportunities to evaluate "nonrevision—called success" conditions. We call this a successful device and application representing in-place and in-function condition at the time of donation. Processing through tissue and organ donation facilities (a partner) facilitates this type of activity (a program started locally in 2005).[7]

Responsibilities for Information Collection and Dissemination

Current local, national, and international guidelines require that retrieval and analysis follow IRB and HIPPA rules and regulations. Although most device retrieval and analysis programs have operated under conditions of information control and nationally standardized procedures, annual review and approval of all participants is now a formal requirement within universities receiving contracts and grants. Our experience over past years is that this component of the studies requires approximately one full-time equivalent of investigator time.

Methods for Three Dental Studies

Three recent dental-oriented activities have been selected for presentation as examples of retrieval and analysis investigations.

Example one: bone implant contact for a root form design

A single design of root form dental implant, that was judged nonrestorable for replacement crowns by one dentist, was removed by surgical trephine, after permission for research study.[8] Approximately 100 single units were removed over 3 years

from this practice site, placed in 10% buffered formalin, and transferred with records for graduate student studies. Stereomicroscopic examinations were used to select 49 candidates where bone along the implant was adequate for midline nondecalcified sectioning. This included Exakt system thin sections, staining with Sanderson red bone stain, and measurement of bone integration using optical microscopy and a Bioquant image analysis system.

Example two: Micro-CT of bone grafts

Patients with edentulous posterior maxillary regions were treated by a sinus lift surgical procedure, which included a calcium phosphate particulate mixed with patient blood as a bone graft.[9] After 30 days, a central region of the implanted bone was removed by surgical trephine to provide a 4×8–mm core as a part of root form dental implant placement. Procedures were done at a single dental office and after approvals; the specimens fixed in 10% buffered formalin were transferred for graduate student studies focusing on micro-CT–based analyses. Specimens were removed from the trephine, oriented for processing, and CT imaged using a university-based micro-CT system. Analysis planes for CT were set at 7- and 20-μm dimensions.

Example three: bone implant contact for a custom osseous integrated implants with particulate bone grafting

Three female patients were treated with implant reconstruction of endentulous mandibles that were subsequently donated for postmortem investigations.[10] Implants were placed in 10% buffered formalin and, with permissions and records, transferred for graduate student studies. After radiographic imaging, six nondecalcified transverse sections were made along left and right distal and along four percutaneous post locations. Nondecalcified thin sections were prepared and analyzed for bone implant contact (BIC) and other bone properties as for the root form devices (discussed previously).[10] These sections were analyzed for nanoindentation hardness properties along the metallic, calcium phosphate–coated, and calcium phosphate particulate (bone graft) interface regions with bone.

RESULTS AND DISCUSSION
History

From the perspective of a university-based program conducting retrieval and analysis studies, the worldwide networking for information and technique exchanges, consensus conferences, and consensus standards has been a valuable

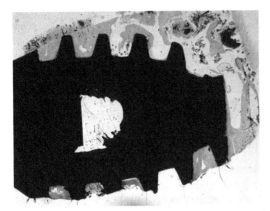

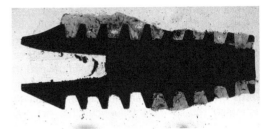

Fig. 2. Midline nondecalcified thin section image of a plateau design root form implant retrieved after 87 months in vivo with a BIC of 59%.

Fig. 1. Midline nondecalcified thin section image of a plateau design root from implant retrieved after 60 months in vivo with a BIC of 52%.

asset. We believe that this approach will continue to benefit all stakeholders.

Conduct of Studies

The process for conducting and reporting of retrieval and analysis investigations has evolved significantly each decade. Currently, many programs exist throughout the world and the value of these types of analyses has been recognized by the profession. Going forward, this area is anticipated to expand as a component of assessing the quality, quantity, and longevity of health care based on surgical implant reconstructive procedures. One intent of the studies on outcomes from procedures using devices constructed from synthetic biomaterials has been to provide a platform of information for future combination and tissue regeneration procedures.

Examples of Dental Implant Studies

The three examples of dental implant studies summarized in this article have been published in part or submitted for journal publication. Therefore, data have been selected to present a brief overview of these types of results, and readers

are referred to the references for more detailed information.

Example one: bone implant contact and histology for a root form dental implant

Examples of the bone, percent bone to implant contact (BIC) and appearance of midline longitudinal images from 5 and 7.25 years are shown in **Figs. 1** and **2**. This particular plateau design implant was constructed from titanium alloy and the surface treatments included (1) roughened by aluminum oxide particulate blasting, (2) plasma spray coating with unalloyed titanium particulate, and (3) calcium phosphate coating. Overall, the percent bone integration was similar for all surfaces (20%–80% BIC) for the 49 trephined specimens with in vivo times ranging from 6 months to 14 years.

Example two: Micro-CT analyses of bone grafts

An example of a midline micro-CT image from one of the 4 × 8 mm cylinder of bone trephined before dental implant placement is shown in **Fig. 3**.

Analyses permitted 3-D quantitation of the bone and bone graft dimensions. Overall, most of the original particulate graft of tricalcium phosphate had resorbed (>80%) during bone healing and the shape-related information showed that regional trabecular bone was progressing to structural maturity (from rods to plate geometry). As discussed in detail within the associated publication, these types of studies provided more quantitative

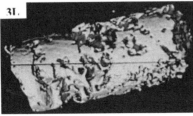

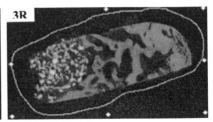

Fig. 3. Micro-CT image from midposition maxillary bone core implanted 12 weeks previously with a tricalcium phosphate bone graft substitute. Images *3L* and *3R* show 3D macro and 2D plane micro-scopic images respectively.

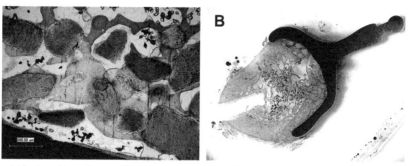

Fig. 4. Nondecalcified section of a postmortem 11-year mandibular implant with alloy and calcium phosphate particulate bone graft, microsection (*left*) and macrosection (*right*).

information compared with our former studies using histologic sections and histomorphometrical data.[9]

Example three: custom-coated implants with particulate grafts

Examples of nondecalcified thin sections prepared from a human donor mandible after approximately 11 years of implant function are shown in **Fig. 4**. Analyses of three similar donor specimens showed osseous integration of calcium phosphate coating, the alloy surface, and the calcium phosphate grafting particulates. These analyses support conditions of longer-term dental function for these types of constructs based on a significant magnitude of bone to implant integration (>30% of surfaces).

EXPERIENCE AND SUMMARY OPINIONS

An overall intent of this summary presentation has been to briefly explain the process of and provide examples from dental surgical implant device retrieval and analysis. Examples of study results have been summarized to demonstrate three areas where unique and new information has been or is being published within professional journals. An analysis of past and current activities strongly supports opportunities for more in-depth investigations of explanted (from revision) and postmortem (en bloc)-type specimens. The coordination of device and procedure registries with focused retrieval and analysis should continue to provide information to enhance clinical outcomes over the next decades. It seems that these types of protocols will be supportive of more fully investigating the clinical applications for successful and unsuccessful outcomes of evolving tissue-engineered medical products as alternatives to some types of synthetic-origin implant devices.

REFERENCES

1. Weinstein A, Gibbon D, Brown S, et al, editors. Implant retrieval: material and biological analysis. Washington, DC: U.S. Government Printing Office; 1981. p. 1–776. NBS Spec Pub. 601.
2. ASTM FO4-561-05, Am. Soc. Test. and Mat. Retrieval and analysis of medical devices and associated tissues and fluids, vol. 13.01. Conshohocken (PA): Annual Book of Standards, ASTM W; 2005. p. 136–51.
3. Retrieval and Analysis of Surgical Implants, ISO 12891-1,3. Geneva (Switzerland): International Organization for Standards; 2007.
4. Schnittman P, Shulman L, editors. Dental implants: benefit and risk, National Institute of Dental and Craniofacial Research/Public Health Service Pub No. 81–531, 1980.
5. Cochran D, Fritz M. Implant therapy I and II. Ann Periodontol 1996;1(1):707–821.
6. Conference Statement and Proceedings, NIH Technology Assessment Conference on improving implant performance through retrieval information: challenges and opportunities. Washington, DC: NIH; 2000.
7. Lemons J. Analyses of in situ and explant surgical implant devices, NIBIB-BRP Grant#R01EB001715, 2005–2010.
8. Lemons J, Anabtawi M, Beck P, et al. Retrieval and analysis of dental implants. J Dent Res, submitted for publication 2010.
9. Chopra P, Johnson M, Nagy T, et al. Microcomputed tomographic analysis of bone healing subsequent to graft placement. J Biomed Mater Res B 2009; 88B(2):611–8.
10. Baker MI, Eberhardt AW, McGwin G, et al. Bone properties surrounding hydroxyapatite-coated custom osseous integrated dental implants. J Biomed Mater Res 2010. Part B – JBMRB – 09–0574 [Accepted].

Index

Note: Page numbers of article titles are in **boldface** type.

Oral Maxillofacial Surg Clin N Am 22 (2010) 425–429
doi:10.1016/S1042-3699(10)00079-8
1042-3699/10/$ – see front matter © 2010 Elsevier Inc. All rights reserved.

Moving?

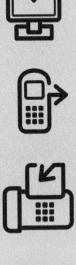

Printed and bound by CPI Group (UK) Ltd, Croydon, CR0 4YY

03/10/2024

01040357-0015